NANCERCIZE!
101 THINGS TO DO ON A
PARK BENCH

*To Stevh,
Let's Nancercize
for life!
Nancy Brig
xo*

Nancy Bruning, MPH

Published by New Moves Publishing
Nancy@Nancercize.net
www.nancercize.net
419-962-6292

An application to register this book for cataloguing has been submitted to the Library of
Congress.

ISBN: 978-0-9856931-0-7
1. Fitness and Health 2. Motivational 3. Exercise 4. Self-Improvement

Significant discounts for bulk sales are available.
Please contact Nancy@Nancercize.net

Book design: Bruce Jacobson
Cover design: Basil Duke

LIBRARY OF CONGRESS PAGE
WITH DISCLAIMER

Disclaimer & Legal Notices

The information provided in this book is for educational purposes only. While the information is based on the latest research and personal fitness experiences, the author is neither a licensed physician nor a health care practitioner and will not be held liable for any damages, real or perceived, resulting from the use of this information. The advice, exercises and tips given in this book are meant for healthy adults only. You must consult your physician to ensure that the information is suitable for your individual circumstances. If you have any physical health issues or any pre-existing conditions, consult with your physician before implementing any of the information provided in this book.

Want to motivate your friends? Share this thought:

"What really makes my day: to feel the wind in my hair and the sun on my skin. To smell the leaves and flowers. To see the greens and blues and every vibrant natural color the changing seasons offer. To hear the birds sing and feel the pleasure and freedom of moving my body in the great outdoors."

TABLE OF CONTENTS

Part I
The Benchmark in Outdoor Fitness

Part II
Stop the 101 Excuses and Do the 101 Exercises

Part III
The Workouts

Acknowledgments

This book would not exist without the enthusiastic support and contributions of "Team Nancercize."

I'll begin at the beginning, with a grateful shout-out to Kevin Jeffrey, who, as then-deputy commissioner of public programs for New York City Department of Parks & Recreation, was responsible for the "Wake Up New York" fitness program that propelled me on the path of outdoor exercise. I also want to extend my heartfelt appreciation to the remarkably capable and dedicated Jennifer Hoppa, Administrator for Northern Manhattan Parks, who unflaggingly promotes physical activity in the parks she oversees. And of course, special thanks to incomparably dedicated and brilliant Parks Commissioner, Adrian Benepe, for all he does for all of us on a daily basis. Another heartfelt thank you goes to New York's Mayor Michael Bloomberg, whose largely unsung but deeply committed work on behalf of New York City Parks has created the climate in which our parks and outdoor exercise could flourish. Imagine if all mayors emulated his PlaNYC goal of a public park or playground within a 10-minute walk of every city resident!

Thanks to the fitness instructors on my Wake Up New York team, who helped plant the seeds and nurtured the concepts that enabled Nancercize to emerge: that wonderful, fun-loving trio—Deliah Barrack, Karen Eubanks, and Ralph Pareda. What good times we had!

My heartfelt appreciation and admiration for those mentors in the public health field who have been my guiding lights. From the New York City Department of Health and Mental Hygiene: Dr. Karen Lee, Director, Built Environment Program, for her creative thinking outside the box; and Dr. Andrew Goodman, Deputy Commissioner, Health Promotion & Disease Prevention, for his faith in parks as an unrecognized partner in health. To Howard Frumkin, Dean, School of Public Health, University of Washington, for his magnificent work in the role of the built environment on health. To Dr. David Sobel, Medical Director of Patient Education, Kaiser Permanente Northern California, who introduced me to the ground-breaking concept of healthy pleasures, of which outdoor exercise is certainly one.

Can you imagine this book without photographs? Neither can I! So, here's to the team of accomplished fitness trainers who demonstrated the exercises and who generously shared their time, talent, muscles, and good cheer: Charles Chadwick, Shawna Emerick, Lisa Priestly, Priest Priestly, and Beth Tascione. And to the photographers who captured it all: Ben Berry, Amala Lane, James Nelson, Roj Rodriguez and Cherie Sprosty.

To the production team who made the book happen: my gifted editor, Judy Katz of Ghostbooksters, with her brilliant understanding of what makes a book speak to its audience; my copy editor Denise Hidalgo, who helped polish the prose; Katz Creative's Wendy Glavin and Basil Design's Basil Duke for their creative book cover and overall design input, and graphic designer Bruce Jacobson for his excellent interior book design and unfailing patience.

I'm also grateful to the friends who read the manuscript at various stages as well as the appreciative and loyal Nancercizers whose constant feedback has pushed Nancercize to evolve; and special thanks to those who helped me "test-pilot" and fine-tune the exercise instructions that appear in the book.

Most of all, I'd like to thank all past, present and future Nancercizers, for their constant inspiration and for their willingness to get up and get out!

An Introduction by Adrian Benepe

New York is in the midst of a green renaissance. Mayor Michael Bloomberg's MillionTreesNYC initiative, launched on Earth Day in 2007, will plant a million trees citywide by 2017 to clean the air, cool the temperatures, and beautify your view. As I write this, we are already halfway there and ahead of schedule. New York City rivers are cleaner than ever, with wildlife returning to the Bronx River and ambitious plans for the Harlem River underway. Each spring millions upon millions of flowers burst into bloom—there are as many flowers as there are New Yorkers.

This wonderful new book by Nancy Bruning puts you in the middle of this promising picture and offers you a new way to see the city around you and interact with it to improve your health and well-being. New York City parks offer you both traditional and surprising ways to energize your day and your outlook. And now, all you need to get started enjoying your favorite spot in a whole new way is a park bench and this book.

New Yorkers are busy people. If they can do four things at once, that's a good thing. With *101 Things to Do on a Park Bench*, they can have fun, get healthy, enjoy the beautiful urban outdoors, and bring the baby or the dog along or get away from it all for a blissful hour.

Want the benefits of a gym workout with no membership beyond being a member of the human race? Step right up. There is no charge for enjoying New York City's outdoor parkland, so forget the excuse of expensive facilities.

Need convenience? There are over 1700 public parks in New York City, so no saying it's too far away.

Wondering where to begin? Nancy's taken care of it.

Nancy is an expert on how to make the most of a New York City park you love, and I applaud her originality and vision. While millions of us have the good sense to occasionally sit on a park bench, breathe in the tree-purified air, and enjoy ourselves, Nancy now takes it to a new and unexpected level. She reminds us that it doesn't take a fancy gym or special clothes or even a warrior's state of mind to get healthy—and happy—in

New York. It's as easy as a stroll in the park with a stop at your favorite park bench.

Adrian Benepe
NYC Commissioner of Parks & Recreation

Part I

THE BENCHMARK
IN OUTDOOR
FITNESS

CHAPTER ONE

Why Nancercize?

Quick—think about that old reliable, taken-for-granted park bench, the mainstay of our public parks and other recreational facilities, not to mention city streets and plazas. See it in your mind's eye. Now, think of things you and other people do on park benches from time to time. What most likely comes to mind are such activities as sitting, reading, snacking, daydreaming, texting, resting, pausing during a run, a bike ride or a walk with your dog—or even sharing a romantic moment with that special someone.

Nothing wrong with those activities! But in this book I'm going to add some new ideas about what you can (and I believe should) do on a park bench. These suggestions may surprise you, will ultimately excite you, and possibly even change your life, as they have for the many "Nancercizers" with whom I have worked.

One thing is for sure . . . after reading this book, you will never look at a park bench in quite the same way.

Here's a question for you: When you think of fitness, what images and sensations come to mind? Might these include weights, treadmills, stationary exercise bikes, germs, bad smells, bright lights, the jarring sound of metal on metal or the blare of your not-so-favorite music over the public speakers? And let's not forget the expense! Not that there's anything wrong with the gym or health club or exercise room—if that's what you enjoy. Confession time: I used to be a so-called "gym rat" (indoor exercise junkie) myself. But, if you're like me and most people, as much as you want to be fit, you don't like those negatives about gyms all that much. So what's the solution?

Well, let's add another element to the equation: Mother Nature. Busy as you are, how much time are you actually spending outside amidst the fresh air, flowers, trees, grass, open sky, and fluffy clouds? Days, weeks, months and even seasons go by, and we intend to get up and out more, as the Parks Commissioner urges us to do, yet most of us, sadly, rarely get out as much as we should . . . not to mention the "up" part. Are you sitting down right now? Have you been outside yet today?

Did I mention there's a friendly park bench in your near future?

It's no secret that, for many reasons (for "reasons" you can also read "excuses"), most of us are not as fit as we want to be—*plus* we don't spend as much time outdoors as we know we should and would really like to.

Also, let's face it, we could be more creative about how we use the resources available to us.

My intention here is to put these thoughts together:
(a) need to work out more to ramp up fitness,
(b) not loving indoor exercise facilities,
(c) need to get out in nature more often, and
(d) park bench as hidden-in-plain sight resource
— and completely change the way you think about an ordinary park bench as well as where and how to get fit!

Connecting exercise with the outdoors and specifically with the ordinary park bench is also an effective way to put fitness within reach of everyone. It does not matter how old or young you are, what your fitness level is right now, how competent or clueless you feel at the start, or how much money you have or don't have … with Nancercize, fitness is completely within your reach. By learning how to use ordinary benches in your local park, your own backyard, on your porch at home or on your apartment terrace (if you are fortunate enough to have one, or a friend with one!) you have all the myriad benefits of a convenient, practical, enjoyable, and totally affordable "workout facility."

As I hope I have now made clear, you will not need a lot of time, fancy workout clothes, or any other exercise equipment, although some people do choose to combine free weights or stretch bands with park benches as a matter of personal choice. With Nancercize, all you really need, though is an open mind, and an inviting, open park bench. (If someone is already seated on the park bench, move to the next one, or better yet, invite them to join you and make a friend!)

I came up with the term "Nancercize" by accident. As a personal trainer and public health professional, I've been designing and leading outdoor exercise programs in New York City parks since 2003. I actually started as a summertime fitness coach for a particular program and expanded to create my own fitness programs in New York City and beyond. One day, as I was walking out of the park after a group exercise session, one of my "fans" quipped, "Why exercise when you can Nancercize!" That struck me as a fun term for what I exhort others to do, and the name stuck.

What I have come to call Nancercize has evolved even further. Today it represents both the philosophy that the outdoor world is our natural health club, yours and mine—and applying that philosophy in our lives by taking advantage of park benches and other objects in our environment and using them to perform a variety of exercises.

To me, everything is fair game for inspiration: calisthenics, yoga, dance, pilates and even martial arts. However, the one common theme, in both my outdoor group classes and with individual clients, is using park benches. The bench is the best tool I've found to create new movements, to make some exercises and stretches easier and safer, as well as to make other fitness movements more challenging.

This book is a reflection of that all-encompassing attitude. Also, with the wide range of exercises, you can easily find those that are individually useful and engaging. It all depends on what you're looking for now and as your fitness levels and energy increase—as they surely will, once you begin to Nancercize!

In this book I have tried to offer something for everyone. By adding a park bench to your fitness picture, a great many exercises that you might have thought were beyond you will suddenly be within your reach. Likewise, a move that has become ho-hum gets a twist that suddenly makes it exciting again. For example, compare Side stretch (#1) to Wishbone (#21); or Modified plank (#64) to Double leg swivel (#74); or Modified push-up (#44) to Handstand push-up (#58). In each case the first is a light effort and the second is a more intense effort. Don't worry—I also provide you with plenty of moderate-level exercises!

Nancercizers range in age from young teens to people in their eighties, and we once had a ninety-something-year-old! Some are affluent, some are of modest means; they are males and females; they exercise solo and in couples—sometimes even a baby or a pet dog joins in. Many of the people I've worked with are total fitness beginners, others are lapsed fitness aficionados, and still others are dedicated exercisers looking for something different to add to their repertoire. What all have in common is their attraction to doing these exercises outdoors. They are also all pleasantly surprised at how easily they can adapt the exercises to their abilities and how effective this simple idea turns out to be.

"But Nancy," you might well ask, "what happens when it rains, or it's too hot or too cold?" And what if you can't get outdoors at all because you're stuck in a hotel at a business conference, or your workplace, with no escape in sight? Or maybe you find the idea of exercising In public potentially embarrassing and feel the need to build up some skill and confidence before you venture outside. Although I'm sold on the outdoors as a great place to be active, I am also a realist. So in this book I also show you how you can do these exercises indoors, on the type of furniture found in offices, homes or hotel rooms. In fact, it is not a contradiction of the Nancercize philosophy but an integral part of it that indoors can be both the place you begin doing these exercises or, at times, the place you use when the weather prohibits you from going outdoors. In any event, when it's time to hit the park where you *really* belong, you'll be confident and looking good.

While Nancercize is a term I use for a particular form of outdoor exercise, the roots of outdoor exercise, sports, and play are ancient and deep. In fact, back-to-nature roots are resurfacing in many exciting forms, including Boot Camp, Parkour, Paleo Fitness's MovNat, GeoCaching, America's Great Outdoor Initiative, and other organized hiking and trail-running groups. Not only in this country but around the world, people are discovering (or better said, *re-discovering*) the joys of nature and the positive effects of being near greenery, sky, birds, and fresher air than you'll find in a gym, home or office.

That's what really makes *my* day: to feel the wind in my hair and the sun on my skin. To smell the leaves and flowers. To see the greens and blues and every vibrant natural color the changing seasons offer. To hear the birds sing and feel the pleasure and freedom of moving my body in the great outdoors. The only thing that gives me the same measure of pleasure is bringing these health-building sensations to other people.

I'm not alone. As I said, this is a growing trend globally. Health professionals are discovering and instructing others on the added mental and physical health benefits of being exposed to nature. Likewise, environmentally conscious urban design professionals are including neighborhood parks in their overall plans. As a result, open spaces are becoming more accessible. Even bean-counting professionals, who study the bottom lines of everything, are waking up to the significant fiscal benefits of making outdoor activity accessible and affordable to the masses. Because people prefer it, or because it's what they can afford, outdoor exercise is becoming the wave of the future. If you want a guide to what types of exercises to do outdoors, how to do them, and also how much to do—well, then Nancercize is for you.

As you will see, I have provided photos and instructions for you for the 101 exercises, based on variations of tried-and-true movements I have used. I have been using them with my group and individual clients for a long time, so I know they work and that they are safe. With these exercises you'll find ways to improve the flexibility, tone, and strength in your arms, shoulders, back, abdomen, legs, and hips. You'll also find exercises that improve your endurance, balance, and coordination. Likewise I give you sample workout routines to follow and use as a springboard for an endless variety of combinations so that your mind and body never get tired of doing the same routine. I help you figure out how much and how often to get exercise, and provide tips on how to integrate fitness into your busy life, or into your current walking, jogging, or bicycling routine. For additional inspiration and clarity there is also a link to a 15-minute video I created which demonstrates most of the exercises. And, I'll be providing more clips on my web site www.Nancercize.net

Most of all, I offer you the freedom of knowing that all you need to get fit is a park bench and an open mind.

Of course it bears repeating this caveat: always talk to your healthcare provider before embarking on this or any new exercise program.

Now let's examine why YOU need to Nancercize....

CHAPTER TWO

Who Will Benefit from Nancercizing?

Here's a quick self assessment. If you identify with one or more of these, Nancercize is definitely for you.

You are a:

Bench Potato: You have a sit-down lifestyle or type of work and need to get up, get out, and take at least a healthy 15-minute exercise and sanity break—for which both your mind and body will thank you!

Gymophobe: You don't like gyms but do want a way to start being more active and stay that way.

Jaded Gym Rat: You love to exercise and are looking for something new that will add variety to your workout.

Aerobic Fan: You have the aerobic walking, running, skating, biking, swimming elements down but are somewhat deficient in the strengthening, flexibility, and balance departments.

Baby Boomer: You need to exercise for health and want to avoid that dreaded middle-age weight gain and layers of body fat creeping up on you.

Savvy Senior: You know you need a gentle form of exercise to keep your sexy shape and allow you to continue to do the things you enjoy doing.

Doctor or Other Health Professional: You realize that you need to have something to offer patients beyond telling them to "get some exercise."

Worried Well: You are at risk for lack-of-exercise-related diseases such as diabetes, heart conditions and osteoporosis.

Managing a Medical Condition: You have been diagnosed with diabetes, heart disease, cancer, or any of the many conditions that exercise and being in nature can help with.

Busy Parent: You want to bring the whole family to the park and get a workout on a bench for yourself while your children get their exercise in the playground. This is an excellent way for you to be a fitness role model for your family, and you may even get some creative ideas from your youngsters for other fun exercises beyond the ones included in this book.

Teen or Young Adult: You think Parkour and free-running are "cool," but you aren't quite up to those activities physically.

Business Traveler/Tourist: You need to keep active while away from home and your regular routine or health club.

Fitness Trainer: You are looking for a way to expand your services and offer your clients something effective but also unique and fun.

Expectant Mother: You want to keep or start exercising, but those crazy hormones are loosening your joints so you need the safety of the bench when you do side-to-side or balancing exercises.

Okay, I trust you now see why Nancercize is, in fact, very much for you, whoever you are . . . so now please turn the page and let's get started!

CHAPTER THREE

Get Ready, Get Set, Get Moving!

I'll never forget my first outdoor fitness teaching job. It was the summer of 2003, in a small park in New York City. I'd been working as a personal trainer for a while to support myself while pursuing a master's degree in public health, and I was involved in a program called "Wake Up New York." At that time I was also the president of a nonprofit organization called The Friends of Fort Tryon Park, and had been writing papers about the health impact of parks, exploring ways to encourage more people to take walks in them.

"Wake Up New York" was the perfect match for me. Four other instructors and I taught three early morning classes, back-to-back. We taught kids or adults, according to our skills. I worked with adults, people of all ages, all of whom had been attracted to this free program that had just been started in their neighborhood park. Although the park had a recreation center we could have used, we all preferred to stay outdoors.

The more we did it, the more the other instructors and I reveled in the freedom of teaching outside the confining box of an exercise room. To make this outdoor exercise program more effective, we developed a new class style—a fluid combination of walking, skipping, lunges, and exercises, using nothing more than gravity and the weight of our own bodies. We used whatever was handy—benches, curbs, and railings—as exercise equipment. The longer we took people on these exercise forays in the park, the happier, stronger, more limber and coordinated, more relaxed and sociable our participants became. As the weeks went by, they felt more comfortable in their bodies and more "at home" working out in the park.

Through word-of-mouth, attendance grew to over fifty people per session—men and women, young and old. People who rarely (or in some cases never) came to the park now came every day, even sometimes taking two or three classes in a row. Others stayed on after class to enjoy basking in the sunshine. Life was great.

With funding for only eight weeks of classes, however, all too soon the program came to an end. During the final moments of that final class, all fifty of us linked arms and formed a closing circle, which had become our tradition in the program. Realizing this was our last day and our last circle, we looked at each other and there were tears.

That was the moment I found my calling: seeing the need to bring basic outdoor fitness to the largest number of people on a continuing basis.

Born to Move
As obviously as we are born to think or eat, we are also born to move. Yet so many of us are missing this crucial ingredient, which is central to living a full, vibrant life.

Take a moment to picture a child running around with his or her pals in a playground, full of joy and glee, and when called to leave, or to come inside from outdoors, for dinner or homework or bedtime, begging for five more minutes of playtime. We've all seen this. Most likely we've lived it.

When did physical activity disappear from our schools, homes, and lives? When did just about everything else become more important than this basic pleasure and need? And even with some of those who do take the time to exercise, how did it become a clock-watching chore, hoping the workout would soon be over?

I pondered these thoughts as I gradually transferred my personal training practice and my own workouts out of the gym and into the park.

For years I had trained myself and my clients indoors, with weights and machines. No question: we got results. I admit I did get plenty of pleasure out of lifting heavy metal objects while staring in the floor-to-ceiling mirrors at my taut body and toned muscles. But over time I also began to realize that workouts don't have to feel so much like work and so little like play. That there don't have to be expensive memberships and fancy equipment. That working out doesn't have to take place indoors under artificial light with the clang of metal on metal and booming music assailing your senses, video screens bombarding your eyes, as negative news clips of world affairs and meaningless celebrity antics ring in your brain. That what I originally thought were "necessities" of fitness were negative aspects that actually get in the way of healthy workouts. One thing that is most telling and reinforces my argument: the majority of those who join health clubs (always starting out with the best of intentions, of course) either never really get started or quickly stop going altogether. We join because this is where fitness happens, or so we think!

Time is another important consideration. It takes time to get to the gym, and once we're there, we want to spend a decent amount of time working out in order to justify the time and effort it took us to get there and get to work or home. So we're often talking about a two-hour commitment, at least. No wonder most of us have a difficult time fitting in fitness.

This is a sad side effect of progress: our jobs and lifestyles no longer require physical movement—and when we want to overcome the difficulties in making time to move more, it is difficult to be as active as we want or need to be. When you make the park your gym, it's likely to be in walking, jogging, or biking distance, so getting there is not only half the fun, it could be half your workout!

According to the Institute for Medicine and Public Health, on average we sit 56 hours a week (that's eight hours per day for seven days)—whether in front of our computers, at our school desks, behind our steering wheels, on a bus or subway, slumped on the couch watching TV. . . commonly it is all of the above and more. Contrast this with the constant movements of our ancestors, and even those three heroic hours (or half-hours) per week on the treadmill that some of us manage, and brag about, become far less impressive.

Sedentary behavior—sitting for long periods of time—is a health risk in itself. Sitting hour after hour literally shuts down your body. Much like an idling computer, your metabolism goes into slow "power-conservation" mode. Your circulation slows, your body uses less blood sugar, you burn less fat, and your risk of heart disease and depression increases. What's more, your spine and back and overall posture suffer. No wonder chronic back pain is at an all-time high. What's surprising is that a one-hour workout three to five times a week, or even running a marathon, does not completely counteract the health effects of sitting down hour after hour. The solution? Taking frequent breaks from sitting such as short walks in the park or up and down the stairs.[1]

Hey . . . even if you're just out for a walk, don't pass by that park bench. . . stop and do a few of my 101 exercises! As you'll see, in addition to full-out Nancercize sessions, these mini-breaks are also perfect opportunities to include Nancercize in your overall health picture.

Why Move Your Body?

Moving our bodies is good for us on every level—physically, mentally, and emotionally.

Regular physical activity can help you to:

- Boost your energy, endurance, and metabolism
- Control your weight and improve your appearance
- Change your brain so it's easier to choose healthier foods
- Tone your body and build strong, lean muscle
- Increase your flexibility, balance and coordination
- Stay younger in body, mind and spirit
- Prevent and manage many diseases and unhealthy pre-disease conditions, including high blood pressure, diabetes, heart disease, osteoporosis, cancer, depression, Alzheimer's and many others
- Improve your mood so that you are better able to handle life's challenges
- Help you sleep better
- Improve your ability to think
- Raise your self-esteem

What's So Special About Outdoor Fitness?

Any physical activity is good for you, but being active outdoors ramps it up a major notch. I know that I am instinctively drawn to nature and the outdoors. Maybe it's my peasant-farmer heritage. But don't we all have outdoorsy ancestors like these from when we were an agricultural society, or even hunter-gatherers, if we go back far enough? According to the Environmental Protection Agency (EPA), indoor air can be from two to a hundred times more polluted than outdoor air. This in itself is a compelling argument for getting outdoors more often. But what compels me as much or more is being in the company of a majestic butterfly, a beautiful budding flower, or even a foraging squirrel. Call me crazy, but I'd rather smell a rose than a locker room. I'd rather notice the seasons changing and feel connected to my environment—even in the winter, even if it's only for an hour—than be shut up in artificial air and light all day long.

Apparently I'm not alone. Evolutionary psychologists tell us that all humans are subconsciously drawn to nature because of our biology. This love of life and living systems has been dubbed "biophilia," and in 1984, American biologist Edward O. Wilson published a book about it. A series of studies recently found that people expect that being outdoors will be more revitalizing than being indoors. So, now you have an explanation as to why we prefer natural surroundings for vacation spots and why we pay premium prices for homes, hotels, and restaurants with a view.

On a practical level, evidence has been piling up for decades that merely being in natural areas such as forests, parks, gardens and beaches restores our bodies and minds [2]. Nature can even help us recover faster from illness and surgery. For example, people whose hospital rooms had windows offering a view of trees and grass recovered better and faster than those in rooms with a view of only buildings or a brick wall. Nature scenes or sounds have helped people control pain, de-stress, and escape.

Compared with a walk on city streets, walking in parks improved scores on memory tests. What's so astounding is that it took very little nature to show this difference—even small parks in urban areas, a potted plant or images of natural scenes had a soothing, health-inducing effect. This potential for better mental health and ability crosses all ages. Richard Louv, in his book *Last Child in the Woods*, coined the term "nature-deficit disorder" to describe what happens to kids who spend too little time in nature; studies have linked nature with improvements in attention-deficit disorder and outdoor play with academic improvement. In his book for adults he refers to a mind/body/nature connection ("vitamin N") that enhances physical and mental health.

It's a lot cheaper to go outside and move than it is to build gyms and a lot of hospitals."
—*Dr. Daphne Miller, family physician, University of California,*
San Francisco,
Quoted in New York Times 11/29/10.

Imagine what might happen if you combine physical activity with being outdoors! Well, researchers are doing just that. A team of American, Canadian, and German researchers found that compared with exercising indoors, "exercising in natural environments is associated with greater feelings of revitalization and positive engagement, decreases in tension, confusion, anger, and depression, and increased energy."[3] They found that exercising outdoors gives us a positive outlook and more vitality— which helps us cope better with all sorts of stressors, including viruses! A study from England suggests that as little as five minutes of exercising in nature is enough to improve self-esteem and other indicators of positive mental health[4]. Is it any wonder that more and more scientists propose that exposure to nature is just as important for our health as exercise and healthy eating?

All natural areas, including urban parks, are considered to be beneficial and green areas, and those with pools, streams, lakes, ponds, rivers or ocean water are even more effective[5]. In fact, we like nature so much that it seems we're more likely to show up for exercise when it's available outdoors, and we're more likely to return for more.

Whether you're frazzled by life and need some soothing and calming, or whether you're tapped out and need some mental and physical revitalizing, nature rocks! Getting your "nature fix" while you get your "fitness" fix is the best kind of multi-tasking.

Why Exercise Outdoors?

According to the National Wildlife Federation, being active in nature is good for us on every level physically, mentally, and emotionally, for both children and adults:

• Enhances fitness
• Restores attention
• Speeds recovery from illness and surgery
• Raises blood levels of vitamin D (which protects against bone loss, heart disease, diabetes, and a slew of other health problems)
• Improves distance vision and lowers risk of developing nearsightedness
• Reduces symptoms of stress and attention deficit hyperactivity disorder (ADHD)
• Improves critical-thinking skills and memory
• Lowers aggression
• Boosts classroom performance
• Sets a good example for our kids

And I would add:
• Meet your neighbors and broaden your network
• Get to know your community and surroundings

Let's Get Started

By now I'm sure you're convinced that outdoor exercise is the way to go. Fortunately, in the Nancercize world, getting started isn't complicated. We think we need lots of time and exercise clothes and high-tech things to move our bodies, but in truth we don't. I've done many of these moves in comfortable street clothes—even wearing a skirt and heels—using benches at bus stops, in city plazas, and so on. I've done them as an hour-long formal exercise session, and I've done just a few of these moves to spark up a walk in the park or as a break from computer watching.

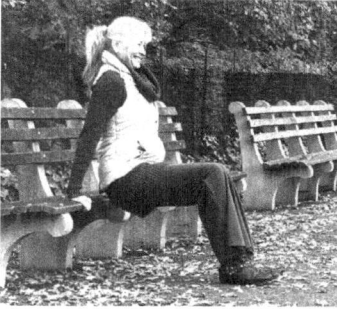

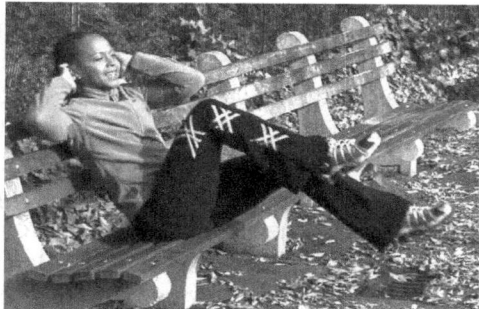

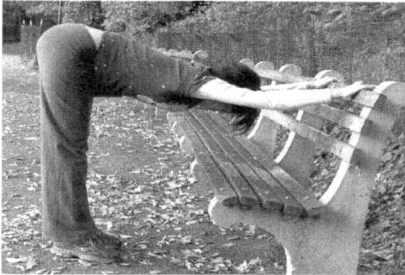

Why not do a few dips or bicycles (#63) or a side stretch, or a table top stretch, while waiting for a bus or your lunch companion to arrive?

Of course, there are recommendations for specific amounts and kinds of exercise, and there's a best way and a not-the-best-way to exercise. If you're not already exercising regularly, these advisories may seem daunting at first. You might think: "How am I going to do an hour a day? Do I really have to think about my breathing?" While an hour a day may be ideal, don't let perfection get in the way of doing something good. If you're completely sedentary now, even 15 minutes a day can make a big difference in your health[5]. And, if you exercise in nature, as I mentioned earlier you can get health benefits in as little as 10 minutes. Experts agree that something is better than nothing. In Part III you'll find templates designed for 5-,10-, 20-, 30-minute and one-hour-long exercise sessions.

How Much Exercise Do You Need? And What Kind?
The American College of Sports Medicine (ACSM), which is the largest sports medicine and exercise science organization in the world, released its recommendations for the quantity and quality of exercise in June 2011.[6] ACSM is the organization through which I am certified as a Physical Activity in Public Health Specialist, so I base my recommendations on

19

their guidelines. According to the ACSM, fitness has four dimensions, as classified by the quality of exercise: aerobic exercise, strength training, flexibility, and—the newest form—neuromotor exercise, which recognizes that balance and coordination are part of total fitness. The 101 exercises in this book are organized into sections that correspond to all these fitness activity categories. As you'll see, using a bench as a prop is especially useful in the newly recognized neuromuscular category because it can help you to improve your balance. Balance has been so badly ignored for so long that many people have trouble with even the simplest basic exercises. Frustration can lead to giving up, which is the last thing you want to do.

Want to motivate your friends? Share this tip:
"If you can't talk while you're exercising, it's too difficult. If you can sing your favorite song, it's too easy!"

Brisk or uphill walking and other aerobic exercises are also an important component of total fitness, and a great place to start. But they are not enough for total fitness, no matter how much of these activities you do. Often we concentrate on one type of exercise because it's all we know or because we are focused on one benefit over the other. We may run or walk on the treadmill or Stairmaster for a long time, thinking it will help us lose weight or prevent a heart attack. And it may. However, other forms of exercise are just as important—and perhaps more important—for heart and bone health, for weight loss, and for body fat loss in particular. For example, when you do it properly, resistance (strength) training builds muscle tissue. This will give your metabolism a boost and help you lose weight more quickly. Resistance training also improves your bone strength and appearance.

Much more so than aerobic exercises, resistance training increases your lean muscle mass. And where health and appearance are concerned, it is your ratio of fat to lean body mass (muscle) that counts. The actual number of calories burned by fat versus muscle is debatable, but health authorities do agree that muscle is metabolically more active than fat. In other words, even when your body is at rest you burn more calories with muscle than with fat[7].

20

In addition, strength training causes microscopic tears in your muscles and, when your body repairs the damage and rebuilds your muscle cells, the "cost" of this process is a higher metabolism. There's evidence that while aerobic exercises raise your metabolism for a few hours after you're done exercising, resistance training can raise metabolism for up to two days. Finally, because a body with a higher muscle-to-fat ratio is toned, taut, sleek, and sculpted, resistance training is the way to go to improve your appearance no matter what you weigh.

Lighten up: Share these with your friends the next time you Nancercize together:
- I like long walks, especially when they are taken by people who annoy me.
- I have to walk early in the morning, before my brain figures out what I'm doing.
- I joined a health club last year, spent about $450. I haven't lost a pound. Apparently you have to actually go there!
- Every time I hear the dirty word "exercise," I wash my mouth out with chocolate.

-- funandfitnessblog

Resistance exercise is for everyone—whatever your age or gender. The truth is, as we age we naturally lose muscle. There is even a name for it: sarcopenia. Our metabolism slows and we become saggy and baggy. Also we can't do as much as we used to—unless we do something about it! As a result, older adults need to do more resistance exercise than younger adults in order to maintain muscle[7]. So, all you boomers who are staving off aging with your cardio workouts, by all means, keep walking, jogging, swimming and biking. But as Elaine Magee, MPH, RD writes on WebMD, "Strength training becomes especially important as we get older, when our metabolisms tend to slow down. One way to stop this is to add some strength training to your workout at least a couple of times a week. The largest muscles (and therefore the largest calorie burners) are in the thighs, abdomen, chest and arms."

Ladies: no need to worry that you'll bulk up too much. It takes a *lot* of weight lifting to look like a bodybuilder! What you *do* need to worry about is not having enough muscle. I've coached many women who are puzzled because they could not seem to lose weight despite spending hours on the treadmill. Adding other forms of exercise, resistance exercise in particular, can make all the difference.

You might have dismissed certain types of exercises because "Those are not for me." For example, you might think of yoga and stretching as ways to relax and not as ways to burn calories or lose weight. Yet studies show that doing yoga to reduce stress, for example, can help take weight off and keep it off, along with many other benefits.

When you incorporate all four types of movement into your life, you are likely to see more of the benefits listed on pages 24 and 28. You're more likely to look better, move more gracefully and do the things you want to do—such as opening a bottle of wine or a jar of peanut butter with a tight lid, bending over to tie your shoelaces, reaching the top shelf, picking up a heavy bag of groceries, rearranging your furniture, remembering the name of a movie you just saw, or even having great sex.

Aerobic Exercise (Cardio)

Aerobic exercise is sustained exercise, such as brisk walking, jogging, cycling, skating, or swimming. These particularly stimulate and strengthen the heart and lungs and improve your endurance. The Nancercize *endurance* exercises are also aerobic. *Strengthening* exercises can be aerobic as well, if you do them with sufficient intensity, speed, and duration, and without long breaks in between sets of repetitions.

Tips:
- Do at least 150 minutes of moderate-intensity aerobic exercise per week. That means 30-60 minutes of moderate-intensity exercise five days per week.
- Alternatively, you can do 20-60 minutes of vigorous-intensity exercise three days per week.
- You may need more—up to 90 minutes of moderate aerobic exercise every day—to lose weight or maintain weight.
- To progress safely and reduce the incidence of injury, gradually increase the intensity, frequency and amount of time of your aerobic activity.
- You can complete your daily exercise minutes in one continuous

session or over multiple shorter sessions of at least 10 minutes each.

Resistance Exercise (Strengthening)
This entails pushing or pulling against resistance, such as weights or machines, exercise bands, or your own body weight. The Nancercize *strengthening* exercises use your body weight, and include exercises for major muscle groups in your lower body, upper body, and core.

Tips:
- Train each major muscle group two or three days each week, using a variety of exercises.
- Very light or minimal intensity is best for elderly people or previously sedentary adults just starting to exercise.
- Wait at least 48 hours between resistance training exercises of a particular muscle group.
- Muscle dictates metabolism—build muscle to boost calories burned, even hours after you've finished exercising.
- If you do multiple reps with light to moderate weights at high speed with few or no breaks, this kind of "circuit training" can also cover your aerobic exercise needs.
- Coordinate your breathing cycle with the movement. Generally it's best to exhale during the most difficult part of the exercise, when you're exerting yourself the most, and inhale during the easier part.

Flexibility Exercise (Stretching)
Stretching exercises improve your flexibility and your range of motion. Nancercize includes many *flexibility* movements.

Tips:
- Do these at least two or three days each week to improve range of motion.
- Flexibility exercises are most effective when the muscles are warm.
- Try very light aerobic activity, strengthening exercises, or a hot bath to warm your muscles before stretching.

Neuromotor Exercise (functional fitness training)
These improve your motor skills, including balance, agility, coordination and gait. They improve physical function, such as walking up or downstairs without using the handrails, or stepping off a curb, can help with everyday tasks such as putting on pants or socks, or even prevent falls.

Many of the *flexibility* and *balance* exercises in this book, including those based on yoga and martial arts, involve this practical type of exercise. Because they are bodyweight exercises, many of the exercises in the *strengthening* and *endurance* categories will improve your neuromotor condition as well. As an extra bonus, the constantly changing outdoor environment forces our nervous system and its connections with our body to learn and grow.

Tips:
- Do these two or three days per week, 20-30 minutes per day.
- Take the opportunity to be conscious of your surroundings and seek out uneven or sloped terrain to enhance your neuromotor skills.
- Dancing also qualifies!

Some Additional Pointers
The ACSM also makes specific recommendations as to the number of repetitions for each exercise or the amount of time you should hold a stretch or do aerobics. I include these here, along with other recommendations that are important for you to know.

For aerobic exercise: One area of debate has to do with aerobic exercise. A technique called "interval training" goes in and out of fashion and is currently popular once again. There is evidence that with this technique you can get better cardiovascular results and quicker weight loss. It's also more fun than just slogging away at the same pace for an hour. Interval training requires you to do short bursts of intense aerobics interspersed with periods of less intense activity. For example, you might start with a five-minute jog, then sprint, do jumping jacks, or do a Nancercize endurance exercise for one minute, then jog again, repeating this cycle several times during your workout. In the Sample Workouts in Part III, I include an example of how this could work with the Nancercize for all three levels of intensity.

For resistance exercise: The ACSM recommends that you do 8-12 repetitions to improve strength and power, 10-15 repetitions to improve strength for middle-age or older persons starting exercise, and 15-20 repetitions to improve muscular endurance. If you're throwing up your hands in frustration at all this counting and keeping track, there is a simpler way. Just repeat each exercise until you can't do any more—a term that is called "muscle failure" or "muscle fatigue." In other words, you can do one "set" of repetitions, rest for a minute or so, and then do another set or two.

For stretching and flexibility: ACSM recommends that each stretch be held for 10-30 seconds to the point of tightness or slight discomfort, and that you repeat each stretch two to four times, accumulating 60 seconds per stretch. Most people think of stretching as "static," where you go into a stretch and hold it steady. While no school of thought advocates actual *bouncing* while in a stretch, there are some approaches that make the stretch more "alive" or dynamic. In yoga, for instance, you breathe into the stretch: you exhale as you stretch into the pose, and, as you inhale, ease up a bit. On the next exhale, you stretch into the pose again, repeating this process several times. There is also dynamic stretching, which I personally love, in which you activate the muscles you are stretching, using isometrics. Whenever possible I'll point out opportunities for making a particular stretch more alive and dynamic.

How to Measure Intensity
The ACSM states that it is best to guide yourself by intensity and time to determine appropriate aerobic or endurance exercise rather than using pedometers, step counters and other devices that measure physical activity, since they are not the best indicators of exercise quality. I agree. Although pedometers or GPS watches are a great reality check on how many steps you are actually taking, a slow walk of 100 steps counts the same as 100 steps of stair climbing, and these are obviously not equal activities. There are many charts and formulas used to determine the desirable heart rate during exercise. I prefer this simple rule of thumb:

• Moderate intensity: Your heart (pulse) rate goes up; you break a sweat; you are still able to talk comfortably.
• Vigorous intensity: Your heart rate goes up substantially; you breathe hard and fast; talking is difficult.

Or:
"If you can't talk while you're exercising, it's too difficult. If you can sing your favorite song, it's too easy!"

Guidelines at a Glance

Type of Exercise	Cardiovascular	Resistance	Flexibility	Neuromotor
Categories of the 101 Exercises	If done in a continuous flow: • Lower Body • Upper body • Core • Endurance	Lower Body Upper Body Core	Flexibility Balance & Flexibility	Balance and Flexibility (and many in other categories)
Frequency	At least 150 minutes/week	At least 2-3x/week	At least 2-3x/week	2-3x/week
Intensity and Duration	30-60 min of moderate 5x/week OR 20-60 min of vigorous 3x/week	2-4 sets of 8-12 reps for strength & power, or 10-15 reps for older persons new to exercise, or 15-20 reps to improve endurance. Light intensity for beginners or older adults. Or, to "failure."	Hold each stretch 10- 30 seconds. Repeat 2-4x to accumulate 60 secs per stretch.	20-30 minutes/day
Progression	Gradual; start with lower intensity after a long break.	Gradual; start with lower intensity after a long break.	Gradual	Gradual
Other Information	Do as one continuous session or multiple 10-min. sessions; interval training may reduce total time needed.	Alternate days for upper and lower body.	Warm up before stretching.	Tai chi, yoga, dancing, are also in this category.

CHAPTER FOUR

Choosing Your Outdoor Gym

Before you begin to Nancercize, you need to prepare yourself by selecting a location. You should choose a place where you feel comfortable and understand how to pick the best bench or benches for your Nancercizing. Parks, plazas, gardens and so on are the best; but in a pinch, you might need to move inside.

Choosing a Location

You can usually find a bench somewhere. I'm fortunate in that I happen to live near (and thus get to work out regularly in) one of the most beautiful parks in the world: Fort Tryon Park in upper Manhattan. But every park, by definition, will give you the gift of nature, including fresh outdoor air, natural light, greenery and other bounties. Some will have water features as well, such as ponds, lakes, streams, rivers or fountains.

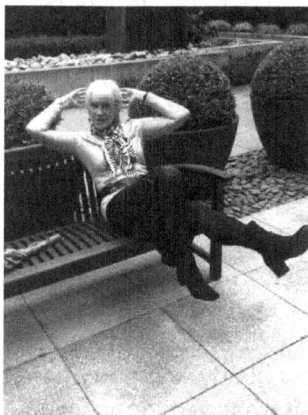

No moment is lost—waiting for my friend to arrive in a plaza in Portland, OR.

Even if your options are limited, you can still be creative and resourceful about what constitutes a workout location. I've Nancercized on street and plaza benches in Portland, Maine; on benches in private gardens and backyards in Holland; along industrial waterfronts and urban lakes in Oakland, California; along boardwalks, bus stops and trolley stops in San Francisco; at the edge of a tennis court in Miami; and on "The High Line" in downtown Manhattan, which is a park created from a converted elevated railroad. There are plenty of other opportunities I haven't even mentioned, such as a backyard, deck, patio, balcony, rooftop – either yours or your exercise buddy's. You could chip in and buy a bench or two and voila—your own outdoor health club. You can get a group together and walk or jog from one outdoor place to another,

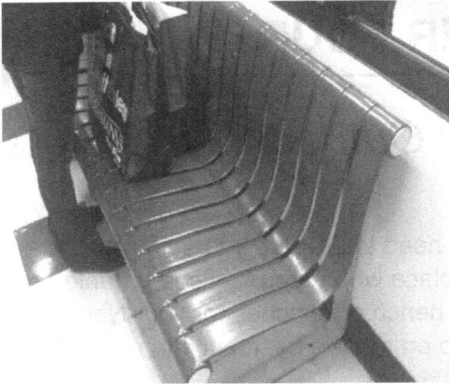

Benches are everywhere—even shopping malls. This one actually has a nice rounded top edge for hand comfort.

using each as an exercise "station." Or how about the grounds of retirement communities, housing developments, sports fields with bleachers, beachfronts and so on? In a pinch, even an indoor or outdoor shopping mall will do, since many of them grant access to walkers before regular business hours and have some bench-like furniture.

Pick a location that you like, one that is convenient, and in which you feel comfortable. Preferably find a location that you can get to on foot or by bicycle, so your "commute" becomes part of your day's activity, and you are already warmed up for your limbering-up flexibility moves. If you can find a place or places with hills or steps, all the better, since that will increase the intensity of your workouts as well as provide a destination or two, perhaps with a view. I find that having a goal like the top of a staircase or a hill is motivating, and so satisfying when you get there!

Does thinking about exercising outdoors—or bravely actually going out and doing it—make you feel a bit self-conscious? Don't worry, this will pass. In all likelihood no one is even looking at you! But you don't necessarily have to do this alone. It does help to have a buddy with you, or be

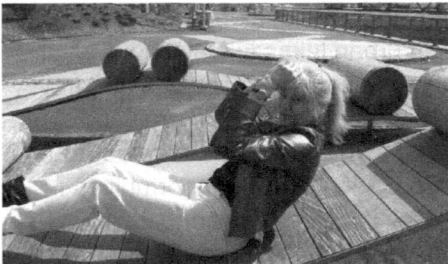

part of a class with others who are doing the same. As you become more adept and self confident, you might actually *want* people to notice you, because then you're helping to spread the word. In any case, taking your spouse, friends or children with you will add to the fun, and allow you to be a role model and motivator for others.

Taking a break from shopping at Ikea in Redhook, Brooklyn.

Choosing Your Benches—and Alternatives

The exercises in this book were designed to be done on an ordinary wooden, iron, or aluminum park bench; even concrete will do. As you may have noticed (or now *will* notice) all park benches are not alike: they vary in design, materials, and location. I've discovered that some exercises feel most comfortable on benches with particular characteristics. For example, push-up- or plank-type exercises, where you rest your hands and body weight on the bench back, will be most comfortable if the bench's back has a rounded top edge. Exercises where you lie flat on your back will be most comfortable if the bench seat is flat rather than rounded in the center or at one side. A flat seat will also be best for most seated exercises so that your backside doesn't perch on either an incline or a curve (see photo below).

The "Tips" section of each exercise gives you the heads-up as to the best bench type for each particular exercise. In the meantime, scope out good locations. If possible, choose a location that has a variety of types of benches—some with rounded back edges, some with flat seats, some with no back, some that have space in front, to the side, or to the back so that you have plenty of room to stand and move. You can put to use bleacher seats in a sports field, and picnic tables with benches also work just fine. You needn't be that fussy. Again, something is better than nothing. When motivated, we humans can be awfully clever in adapting to almost any situation. Just watch out for splinters on those old wooden benches!

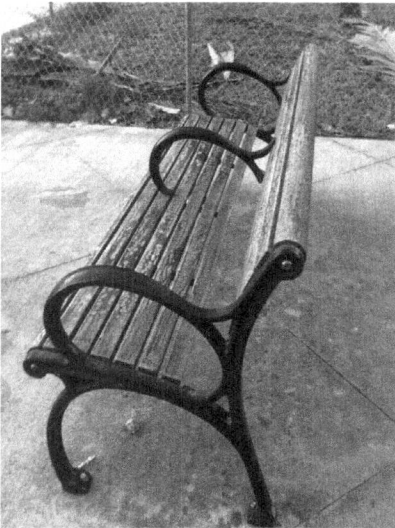

Outdoor Alternatives

If, for whatever reason, you are not able to utilize a park bench, you can adapt the exercises to other park features. I rarely see a wall, railing, curb, step—you name it—that I can't use

Meet the bench, your new best friend. Seek out benches with a rounded back edge and a flat seat. They make many of the exercises easier and more comfortable.

29

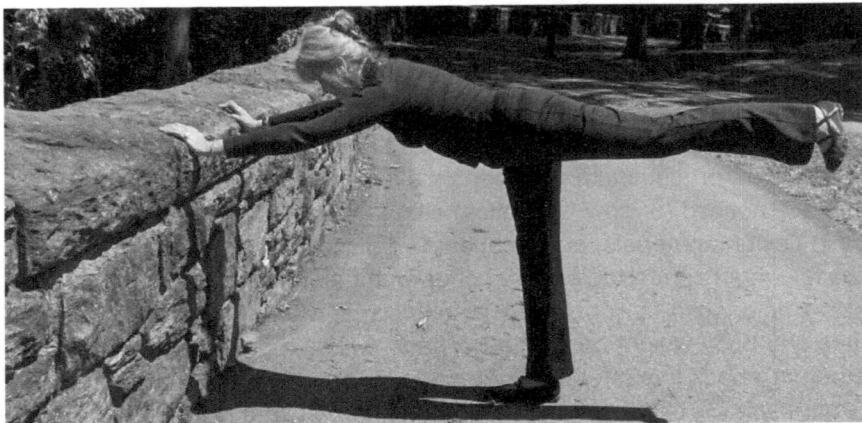

Depending on your location, you might use another park feature instead of a bench. I use walls, or railings in addition to benches.

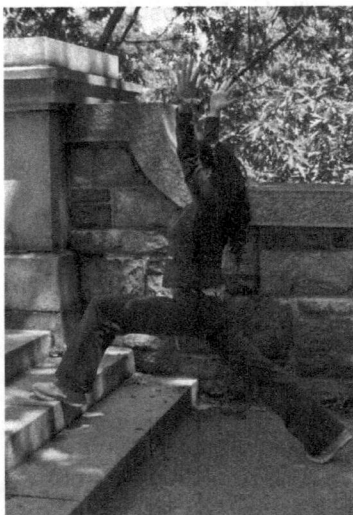

A low curb can be a great alternative to a bench, too.

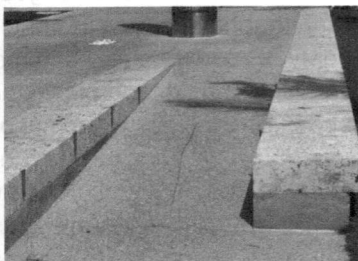

Is this a bench or a curb? Doesn't matter—we can use it to Nancercize.

as a prop for exercise. Once you're in Nancercize mode, you'll see the world with new eyes. Some of my longtime clients are so well trained that every time they see a bench or other exercise-friendly outdoor feature, they feel a strong urge to do some push-ups, dips, or stretches. The world can be your health club, too—experiment!

Indoor Alternatives You can do these exercises indoors, too! Say you're traveling and stuck in a hotel room, conference room, or at the office, and could use a break—even a fast one. Or you might be practicing at home, even reading this book, preparing yourself to go outside to Nancercize. It might be raining, or cold, or hot, or there might not be a park around.

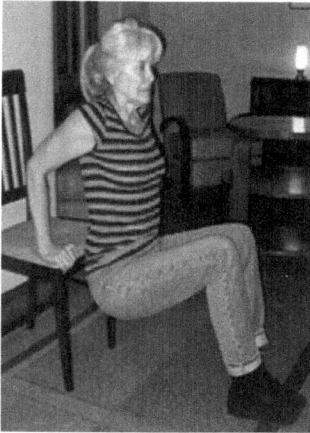

Bad weather? Stuck in your hotel room? Do your Dips on a chair.

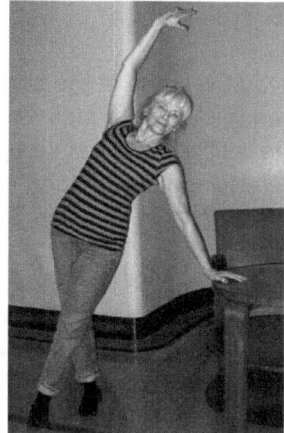

A coffee table works just fine for a Side Stretch; so might a counter top or desk.

Whatever the reason, look around for furniture that serves the same purpose as a bench. It has to be sturdy, about the right height for you, and allow you enough room to perform the necessary movements.

For example, you can do many of these exercises using a regular (but sturdy!) chair—just make sure to push it up against a wall so it doesn't shift or slide when you perform the exercises. You can sometimes use a tabletop, counter, or desktop. You can also use a sofa or bed, or perhaps a coffee table if it is the right height. Again, make sure nothing is going to shift when you use it. For some exercises, you can also use the floor.

Bodyweight Exercise with Benches

The resistance exercises in this book are bodyweight exercises—the resistance is provided by your body rather than barbells, dumbbells, medicine balls, kettlebells, elastic bands, or other equipment. Bodyweight exercise is fitness in its most basic form . . . it's just you playing against gravity. Those "old school" calisthenics for example—push-ups, sit-ups, squats—those are bodyweight exercises, and they've withstood the test of time as great body conditioners.

Bodyweight exercises have the added advantage of requiring more flexibility and balance to perform the movements; as a result they work more parts of the body. I've arranged the bodyweight exercises into categories such as flexibility and upper or lower body strength. However, what you are really doing is working more of your body and in more ways no matter which category you're in. The category headings in this book only tell

31

you the parts of the body that are particularly affected by that specific exercise. Another plus to bodyweight workouts is that when you do many repetitions without stopping, or with just a brief rest in between, you're increasing your endurance and working your heart and lungs in the same way aerobic exercise does.

Some people are under the mistaken impression that bodyweight exercises are either too difficult, or in some cases, too easy for them. Nothing could be further from the truth—they are infinitely adaptable to whatever your fitness level.

When you work out on and with a bench you can make an exercise easier or more difficult, depending on where you place your weight and which muscles are involved. In physics, this is called *leverage*. For example, you can make a basic push-up easier by placing your feet on the ground and your hands on the bench back or seat. The steeper the angle of your body, the more the leverage factor is working in your favor, in effect, making your bodyweight lighter. Or you can make a push-up more difficult by placing your feet on the bench and your hands on the ground. In this case, the angle of leverage is working to make the exercise harder because gravity is effectively increasing the amount of bodyweight supported by your arms.

I've indicated the level of difficulty for each exercise, from light to moderate to intense, and have given you various versions, modifications, and tips to bump the level up or down. In the Tips section of each exercise, look for a (+) plus sign if you want a more challenging version; look for a (-) minus sign for a less challenging version if you need that. You can experiment on your own as well—instead of adding or subtracting weight as you would in a gym, you adjust the angle of your body in performing the movement. For many women this is especially useful because they often feel they need to start working their upper body with light weights, and therefore they consider bodyweight exercises too difficult. But if an exercise is, in fact, too difficult for you to do at first, you can use leverage to make the exercises easier for yourself. At the other end of the spectrum, plenty of highly seasoned professional athletes and "boot camp" military-style trainers use "advanced bodyweight exercises," so they can be modified to be challenging for even for elite athletes in peak condition.

CHAPTER FIVE

Identifying the Exercises That Are Right for You

The bench exercises in Part II are meant to complement aerobic exercise such as walking, jogging, cycling and so on. As I said earlier, an aerobic or cardio workout enhances your heart and lungs while it improves your endurance, ability to handle stress, and sleep patterns. This is all good. However, cardio workouts usually emphasize the lower body. What about the rest of you? The strengthening, flexibility, and balance exercises I include, all of which have stood the test of time, will help ensure that you are able to work your entire body in several ways. While elliptical and rowing machines as well as Nordic walkers do include the upper body, your movements are limited to one direction, or plane. Nancercizing, as you'll see, works your entire body in multiple directions and planes, enlivening and challenging your muscles, bones and joints as nature designed them to be.

Watch the Video
In either case, you may want to start by watching my video, *101 Things to Do on a Park Bench*. Just go to my website, www.nancercize.net, and click on the video link on the Home Page. Watch it all the way through to familiarize yourself with the exercises, and for inspiration. Once you've decided which exercises you initially want to do, you can always go back and review specific exercises. Visit Nancercize.net for short instructional clips of these and new exercises, too.

Decide on a Level
Your next step is to choose a level of exertion. I've rated each exercise as either light, moderate or intense. I'd recommend that everyone start with light exercises, at least the first time around. If you've been rather sedentary and are just beginning, definitely go with "light." You should also "go light" if you're pregnant or recovering from an illness or medical treatment. Better to be safe than sorry. You may surprise yourself as to

what you can do, and what you can't actually do, especially if you have been doing an exercise using incorrect form (more about that later). As you progress, you'll be able to do additional repetitions of each of your chosen exercises and move yourself up to the next level of intensity. But please, be patient with yourself. It's a cliché that rings true: Rome wasn't built in a day. Neither are biceps.

Also, research shows that some new habits can take a couple of months to become ingrained. Stick with Nancercize for at least a month or two and be surprised at where it takes you!

Choose Your Exercises
The exercises and stretches included were inspired by tried-and-true, old school calisthenics, Yoga, Pilates, martial arts, and dance. The unifying factor is that all are modified to be done utilizing a bench or the like, sometimes to support you in exercises you might find to be too much of a challenge without the bench, and sometimes as a way to make exercises more challenging. Many of them can be done while sitting, so if standing is one of your limitations, you can still use the bench exercises. No matter what your condition or your fitness goals, you'll find something here for you!

Let's say you have never have been able to do a push-up, and you don't want to modify it the usual way by putting your knees on the ground. No problem! Simply place your hands on the bench back or seat as in #44—and voila!—push-ups are within your reach.

Or, at the other end of the spectrum, let's say that push-ups have gotten too easy—in fact boring—for you. Again, no problem! Try the One-Armed Power Push-Up (#56), the Push Off and Clap (#48), or the Push off and Clap (#58) or Handstand Push-Up. I guarantee your boredom will vanish as you rise to the extra challenge.

Perhaps certain stretches, such as a backbend, have been too scary for you up till now. With Nancercize, instead of the classic yoga version done on the ground, you will bend only half as far with your hands on the bench (#97). If you've ever done yoga with props, think of the bench as a great big supportive yoga block that you don't have to buy or carry around. Same thing for exercises that require balance or coordination.

34

The bench provides you with support and prevents injury—for example in the Triangle Pose (#87) and Seated Sun Salute (#100).

A Smorgasbord of Delicious Choices for Every Occasion
Think of this book as a menu of movements. You can choose exercises from each category to assemble a whole-body workout (a "banquet"). Or when you're really short on time or just taking a break from sitting too long, choose one or two quick moves (a "snack"). You could decide to do one or two of the exercises on your way during a casual walk in the park, before a meeting in your hotel room, at home during a commercial break on TV . . . well, you get the idea. I've spent many a "wasted" moment waiting for an elevator or while yakking on the phone also doing squats, balances, or push-ups against a wall. Not to mention the literally count-less Nancercize "snacks" I've had while writing this book! Unlike food snacks, tidbits of Nancercizing throughout the day will help you whittle the weight down, not cause it to creep up.

Your own 5-, 10-, or 15-minute Nancercize snacks a day can add up to an entire meal by the end of the day. And, as I explained earlier, being active for short periods throughout the day may help solve the health problems that come from sitting hour after hour—in ways that even long three-times-a-week workouts don't. As an added bonus, you also won't get all sweaty!

Follow the Leader or Create Your Own
You can either follow the workouts I've provided in Part III or create your own. If you are new to exercise, I recommend that you begin with the pre-designed workouts. Then you can, if you like, gradually modify them by switching out certain other exercises in the same category. Since the number of combinations of exercises is infinite, you should never get bored!

CHAPTER SIX

Putting It All Together and Making the Best Use of This Book

Remember that these exercises are meant to complement whatever aerobics you're doing: I personally prefer to have my clients do intense aerobics toward the end of the workout period; I don't want people to become so tired that their form suffers. You may prefer to do your aerobic workout first, or interspersed throughout, as I describe in Circuit Training, below. If you do all-out aerobics first, be sure to taper into light aerobics before you begin to do the flexibility exercises, and pay particular attention to your form.

Full Body Workout If you are on an every-other-day schedule, you can strengthen all three body areas during your workout for a full body workout. Start with a warm-up of light aerobic exercise—for example, walking to the park, or walking around the park for 5 minutes. Then do one or more flexibility exercises, which will loosen up and lubricate your joints, increase blood flow, and wake up your mind and body. Then proceed though a selection of strengthening exercises, working the large muscles of your lower body, the smaller ones in your upper body, and the support muscles in your core. If you're not doing enough aerobics or if you just want to spice up your routine, add some endurance exercises from that category. Finish off with the balance and flexibility moves. Just be sure to include one or more exercises from each category to guarantee you get the recommended amount of all four types of exercise. Doing this will strengthen all three areas of your body. And again, please remember to choose the right level for you and, as you become more fit, allow yourself to progress to the next higher level.

General Plan You can use this general plan to create your own customized workouts. The time frame for each component depends on the total length of your workout. For specific guidelines, see the 36 sample workouts provided in Part III. If you'd like to see more workout ideas, visit my website nancercize.net and subscribe to my newsletter. If you have questions, email me at questions@nancercize.net

- Light aerobics to warm up
- Flexibility exercises/loosening up
- Strengthening exercises: lower body, upper body, core
- Endurance exercises or Aerobics
- Flexibility & Balance exercises to cool down

Upper or Lower Body Workout If you are working out every day, follow the same general plan as outlined above, but don't do strengthening exercises for the same body area two days in a row, especially if you are working your muscles to the point of fatigue. So, if for example you do upper body on Monday, do lower body on Tuesday and upper body on Wednesday, and so on. You can do Core, Flexibility, Balance and most Endurance exercises every day if you like.

Try a Circuit You might prefer to do all your exercises at one stop on your walk. I prefer to intersperse them with brisk walking. I think of this as a simple circuit-style workout. We do some brisk walking, then warm up, then walk some more, then do a lower-body strengthening exercise, then walk some more, then do an upper-body strengthening exercise, walk some more, do some core work, do a brisk or uphill walk and/or endurance exercises, then cool down with balance and flexibility exercises. In a small park we might walk around the park several times, repeating the circuit. In a large park we do one long circuit. The distances we do for aerobic walking depend, in part, on the location of the exercise "stations." In some parks you might stop where you have the best views. In other parks the type and condition of the benches influence where you stop to exercise.

You can repeat the same workout for a couple of weeks, increasing the repetitions and intensity of the individual exercises as you progress. When you're ready, you can create a new workout from the menu, using the same principles.

Use Good Form Now I'm going to talk about something that's very important—form. Form is a specific way of performing a movement. You need proper body position and alignment to get the most out of your effort, to prevent injury, to make sure you're actually using the muscle or muscle group you're aiming for; and finally, to prevent cheating. Actually there's one more thing: It looks and feels better! Where's the pleasure (or the best use of your time and body) of doing something in a sloppy way? I'm a stickler for doing the exercises precisely and correctly—ask anyone I've worked with! Often I'll see someone working out on their own in the park, and their form is all wrong. I'll joke with my clients that I hope the person marries an orthopedic surgeon, because they'll need one—but it really is no joke. Even if you think you know how to do an exercise, please do read the instructions, look at the photos, and watch the video. I give you tips on what to watch out for in each exercise so you will use great form and achieve your desired results.

The most common things I see happening are:
- Your chest collapses inward and your shoulders hunch forward or creep up towards your ears. Correct form usually means keeping your shoulders down and back, with your chest open.
- Your head falls forward or your chin juts out. Generally, you want to keep your head and neck in line with your spine.
- Your abdominal muscles are inactive and just hanging out. Instead, keep them contracted and engaged as if you were pulling your belly button to your spine. This allows your lower body to align properly.
- Your chest sticks out in front and your butt sticks out in back, like an S-curve. Best solution is to gently drop your tailbone down, and simultaneously imagine a thread pulling you upright from the top of your head. This double move automatically helps you straighten up and engage your core muscles to support your posture.

To become familiar with the correct way to do the exercises, I suggest that you practice them at home. If a big mirror is around, use it to check your form. Whether you begin at home or at a park, focus on the quality of your movement rather than merely on the quantity of repetitions. I'd rather you did three slow perfect push-ups than 25 fast ones using poor form. Build up gradually to more (perfect) repetitions.

Buddy Up I highly recommend that you do the exercises with a buddy, especially at first. You can both look at the photos and video to get the gist, and then one can read the instructions as the other does the exercise, and vice versa. Or get a Nancercize group together for socializing and networking. I think all the exercises are more fun when you have a partner, but look for opportunities to add an extra, playful dimension. For example, when doing Thread the Needle (#78) do it back to back with your buddy and, when you reach through, tap each other's hands. I guarantee it will make you smile. Too, it helps to have people around to check each other's form. If possible, work with a trained professional, especially at first, to help you do the exercises correctly. Plus, you'll probably feel more brave and less self-conscious when you have other people around you doing the same thing. There's an old saying to the effect that "When one person does something new, they're crazy, when two people do it, it's normal, and when three or more do it, it's a movement."

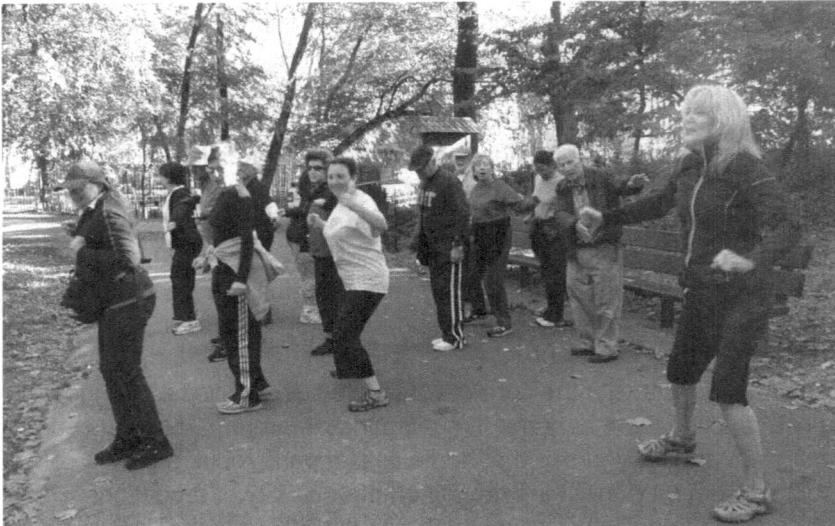

Let's get moving!

Common-Sense Safety Tips

- If you have a chronic disease or disability, talk to your doctor before beginning.
- Build up to activities gradually, especially if you have been inactive.
- Move slowly into a position; never jerk or "lock" your knees or elbows.
- Coordinate breathing with your movements.
- Warm up and cool down with light activity such as walking.
- You should feel your muscles working, but you should never hurt.
- If you feel exhausted, or have sore joints, unpleasant muscle pulling, dizziness or chest pain, you're overdoing it.
- Drink plenty of fluids, especially in hot weather, and stop exercising if you exhibit signs of overheating such as dizziness or nausea.
- If you are exercising in cold weather, dress in layers, and come inside when your fingers or toes begin to feel numb.
- Be alert and aware of your surroundings at all times; avoid wearing ear phones.
- Exercise with a buddy or two if possible; outdoors, stay on well-traveled, well-lit paths if you are alone.

We Brake for Wildlife: A Whistle Pig? In New York City?

One of the great pleasures of outdoor exercise is the chance to see a variety of animal life. Even in the most developed city, there are critters sharing the space with you—most likely birds, but be on the look out for other animals too. I've seen eagles, hawks, vultures, cardinals, orioles, crows, blue jays, seagulls, and hummingbirds to name a few. I've seen ground hogs (aka wood chucks or whistle pigs), skunks, squirrels, chipmunks, and even an opossum one morning. I use my iPhone apps to help me identify them, and often write about them in my blog, on the Nancercize Facebook page, or in my newsletter. So, please visit nancercize.net, like facebook.com/Nancercize, and subscribe at Nancercize.net and prepare to be delighted with the unexpected.

Let's Talk Weather

One of the first things people ask me about outdoor exercise is, "What about heat, cold, rain and snow?" I say, "Go for it anyway—but be smart and be prepared." Light rain or snow is easy to deal with—wear your waterproof gear for the walking or running part of your outing, and seek out sheltered places to do your Nancercizes, such as beneath an awning, in an outdoor pavilion, on a pathway under a bridge overpass or in a park tunnel. Some of the most enjoyable park times I've had were during a soft rain or a gentle snow. Under those circumstances we just stick to standing exercises rather than sit down on a wet bench. Cold and heat are also manageable, provided you follow the tips below. And of course have a Plan B in place: If the weather is unbearable, don't use that as an excuse to remain on your couch. Surely you're smarter than that! Just use your indoor furniture instead of a bench. An indoor workout now and then will increase your appreciation of the time you get to spend outdoors!

Cold Weather Tips Okay, I admit it: I hate cold weather. But I love winter—the outdoors is so beautiful, despite the lack of leaves. Remember the beautiful aspects of winter: tree limbs silhouetted against a brilliant blue sky; spectacular winter sunsets; the soft silence of snowflakes floating to the ground and the satisfying crunch of crystallized snow under your feet.

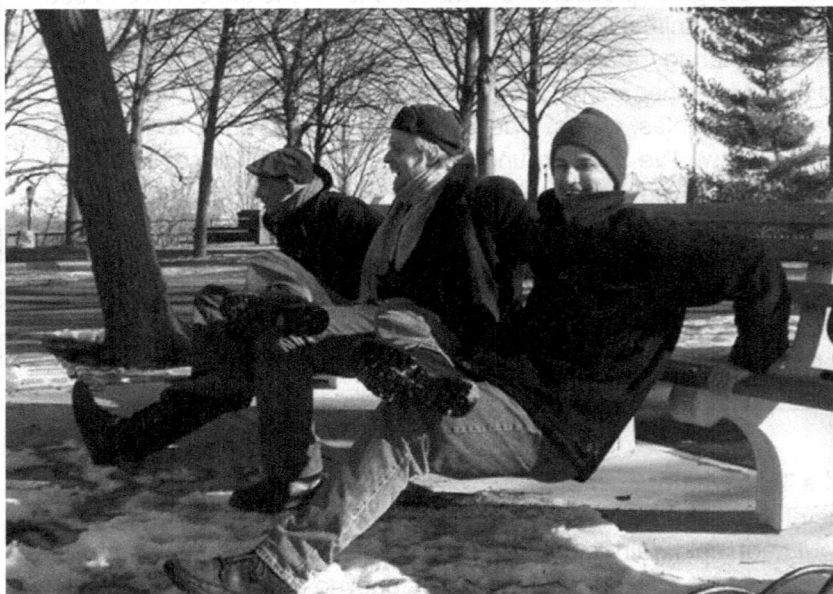

Neither rain, nor snow, nor lame excuses like cold weather will keep us from doing our Nancercizes.

It's all too easy for us to use the cold as an excuse for staying indoors. But a recent study in *Obesity Reviews* suggests that staying indoors where it's toasty warm may be adding to our overweight problems—and not just because we're more sedentary. Avoiding exposure to colder temperatures reduces the calories we burn and diminishes our ability to generate heat when we need it.

How then does someone like myself who leads fitness walking groups in the winter survive? I've learned a lot in the seven years I've been leading the Fitness Walks. Mostly you need to dress for the occasion. Here's what experts recommend to stay warm: the goal, according to the American College of Sports Medicine, is to "generate and maintain a warm air pocket close to our body."

1. Dress in layers. (This one's a no-brainer!) Although I look back fondly on my youth in Brooklyn, when we dressed in thick, heavy playsuits that left us waddling like the roundish people in the Disney film *Wall-E*, I bless modern technology. Three or more thin layers are better than one or two thick ones.

2. Modern miracle fibers such as thin polyester and polypropylene are best, especially for the inner layer, since they are lightweight, do not readily absorb moisture, and wick moisture away from your skin. This insulates you even when you sweat.

3. For workouts, natural fibers, sadly, are not so good. Avoid wool or cotton since they absorb moisture easily and become heavier and bulkier when wet. An exception that might be good for some people is to wear polypropylene on the inside and thin wool socks on the outside to keep your toes toasty.

4. Fluffy is a big no-no! Avoid down and pile clothing since they can overheat you and cause excessive sweating.

5. Add a liner. Invest in a pair of thin polypropylene glove liners or socks. Remember, too, that mittens are warmer than gloves.

6. Waterproof wisely. When it's wet out, add a waterproof outer layer, preferably with vents to let out the heat and humidity your body will

produce. Accumulating moisture inside your shell is a recipe for hypothermia.

7. Keep a lid on it. Cover your head with a hat or headband made from windblock fleece—this allows sweat to evaporate while blocking the wind.

8. Stay loose. Avoid tight clothing, which hampers your circulation.

9. Don't forget your eyes. Protect your eyes from bright or reflected sunlight and from the cold wind and make sure your sunglasses are UV-safe.

10. Use common sense when ground conditions are dangerous. I often will take an alternate route to avoid icy patches on the path, or slippery wet leaves on a downhill slope.

More Cold Weather Tips
- Breathe through your nose to moisten the air before it hits your lungs.
- Cold, dry air can make the air passages in your lungs constrict, causing feelings of chest tightness or persistent dry cough (even if you don't have asthma).
- Drink plenty of water even if you don't feel thirsty—dry winter air can increase your water loss through breathing.
- Protect your skin with a good moisturizer and your lips with lip balm.
- Consider using chemically activated hand and foot warmers.
- And for goodness sakes, come in out of the cold when you start to shiver and your fingers turn blue!

Hot Weather Tips Do you know that old saying, "Only mad dogs and Englishmen go out into the noonday sun"? As clichéd as it might sound, that idea is a great place to start being smart about outdoor activity in warm weather. Rule # 1: Don't go out during the hottest part of the day. But there are other points to consider as well, whether you want to Nancercize, participate in a pick-up basketball game, play tennis, have a jog or just take a walk.

First, let's have a little science lesson on how hot weather affects your body. Exercising in the heat puts extra stress on your body—especially those vital organs known as your heart and lungs. Exercise itself raises your temperature and the air temperature adds its own heating effect. To handle the load, your body pumps more blood through your skin. Unfortunately this means there's less blood for your muscles, so to compensate your heart will beat faster.

Another popular saying is "It's not the heat—it's the humidity." That's even truer when we're exercising! If the humidity is high, your body is extra-stressed because your sweat has a harder time evaporating from your skin. Losing this natural cooling effect raises your temperature even higher.

Tips for Keeping Cool
Following these tips should keep your bodily "mechanics" running smoothly. If you have a chronic medical condition or take medication, don't neglect to ask your doctor if you need to take additional precautions.

1. Easy does it. Start slow, and as your body adapts to the heat, gradually increase the length and intensity of your workouts.

2. Drink up. You need to be hydrated for your cooling system to work. Drink plenty of water while you're active, whether you actually feel thirsty or not. Some experts recommend sports drinks if you'll be exercising more than one hour. These drinks are meant to replace the sodium, chloride and potassium you lose through excess sweating. But by all means avoid caffeine or alcohol because they can dehydrate you.

3. Keep it loose. Stick to lightweight, loose-fitting clothing because they promote sweat evaporation and cooling by allowing more air to pass over your body. Those who live in New York and love to wear black clothing year-round (me too, guilty as charged!) may find it difficult to follow the standard advice to avoid dark colors because they absorb more heat than light-colored garb, but this is important advice.

4. Time it right. Exercise in the morning or evening—when it's likely to be cooler outdoors—rather than in the middle of the day. And know when

it's time to call it quits . . . preferably before symptoms of heat stroke appear!

5. Wear sunscreen and a hat. If possible, exercise in the shade. Sunburn is no fun, and it also decreases your body's ability to cool itself.

Watch Out!
Your natural cooling systems may fail if you're exposed to high temperatures and humidity for long periods. The resulting heat-related illness causes heat cramps, heat exhaustion or heat stroke. Take it from me, these are no fun. The first summer I led fitness classes in a New York City park (three classes, back to back, at the height of the summer) I spent most of that time with three or more of the following symptoms of heat illness:

• Weakness
• Headache
• Nausea or vomiting
• Loss of appetite
• Rapid heartbeat
• Dizziness
• Muscle cramps

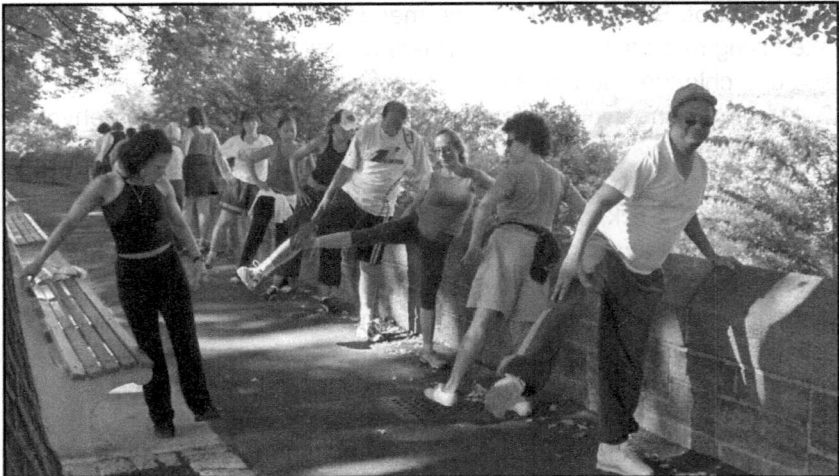

Take advantage of shade if possible to keep cool and avoid getting too much sun.

The Mayo Clinic recommends the following: If you show signs of a heat-related illness, stop exercising and get out of the heat. Drink water, and wet and fan your skin. If you don't feel better within 60 minutes, contact your doctor. If you develop a fever higher than 102 F (38.9 C) or become faint or confused, seek immediate medical help.

A Word about Sunlight

Spending time outdoors increases our exposure to sunlight. Before you run for cover, listen to this: it is believed that sunlight deficiency is linked to a high incidence of irritability, fatigue, illness, insomnia, depression, alcoholism, and suicide[8]. Sunlight is healthy! Once sunlight reaches your eyes and is registered by the brain, your entire body is affected in a positive way. We depend on the energy of sunlight to catalyze many processes in the body, including our ability to burn fat and get rid of toxins. Research by photobiologist John Otts suggests that this is true of full-spectrum natural sunlight only, not partial sun. In addition, studies indicate that we as a nation—because of all the time we spend indoors these days—are experiencing a mass vitamin D deficiency (there's a simple blood test you can take to see where you stand). Age, obesity, dark skin, and illness increase your risk for this deficiency, as does living in the Northern part of the country or if you are a sun-phobe or a sun-block lover. Vitamin D deficiency is also linked to osteoporosis and rickets in children, plus hip fractures, autoimmune disease, several types of cancer (including skin cancer), diabetes, cardiovascular disease, and depression[9].

Sunlight is the main source of vitamin D for humans. This, for me and for many other concerned public health professionals, is another reason to get outdoors when we exercise. However, this doesn't mean that we can hang out in strong sunlight for hours on end. According to integrative physician Dr. Frank Lipman, as a general rule if you are not vitamin D deficient, about 20 minutes a day is adequate in the spring, summer and fall without sunscreen on your arms or legs. In the winter the sun is not strong enough to generate enough vitamin D north of 37 degrees latitude (the latitude of San Francisco) no matter how long you're outside[10].

A few safety rules apply. Never, ever stay out long enough to get a sunburn. You need to be especially careful if you have fair or sensitive skin or a personal or family history of skin cancers, or if you are taking medication that makes you sun sensitive. It is preferable to go out in the early morning or later in the day when the sun is weak or has gone down. Wear protective clothing if you can't avoid too much sun.

I also suggest that you seek out tree-shaded benches or those under a gazebo. I've seen great gazebos and shade pavilions in Florida, where the sun is strong all year round. In winter, in climates far from the equator, most people don't need to worry, but if you live in or visit the southern latitudes, ask your dermatologist to recommend a nontoxic brand of sunscreen.

Sunlight's benefits make sense because we evolved in the sun; we were made to get some sun, not to live our lives indoors or have to coat ourselves with sunscreen every time we go outside. Remember also to take antioxidants when you sit in the sun, as these can help protect skin cells from sun damage.

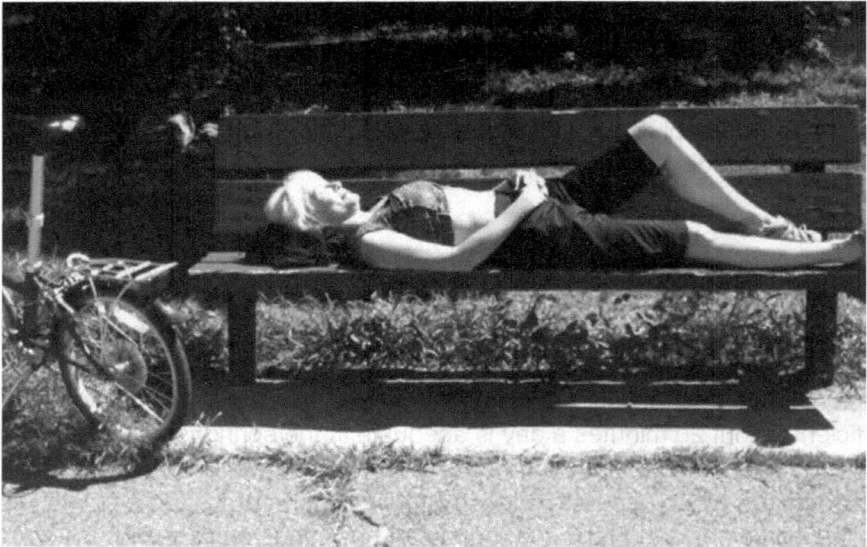

Sometimes a bench is just for relaxing.

CHAPTER SEVEN

Making Outdoor Fitness a Regular Part of Your Life

Nancercize, for me, as I said at the beginning of this book, is the philosophical belief that all outdoors is our natural "health club." One part of what I do professionally is to coach, motivate, teach and lead people in the best possible ways to not only get fit and healthy, but also how to enhance their quality of life, day by day. And if you actually stop to smell the flowers—in other words, be fully present in all the moments of your daily life—your life will never be the least bit dull or boring. Wonders lie all around us, and often we are too distracted to see what is right in front of our eyes.

And speaking of *being present,* have you ever heard this:

The past is gone; forget it.

The future is unknowable.

But this moment is a gift.

That's why they call it *The Present.*

Nancercize then, is more than my "business." It is my passion. Even more than that, it is a movement I want to start, nationwide, perhaps even worldwide.

Hey, if I am exhorting you to be outrageous and think outside the box when it comes to exercise, why shouldn't I also dream big!

Just getting outside and seeing how good it feels may be enough to keep some individuals on a regular "get up and go" cycle. I am all for whatever will make the 101 exercises included in this book personally meaningful to you and act as a strong motivator. Let me just add this: besides feeling and looking better, my Nancercizers report such benefits as being an infinitely more patient partner, parent or friend, enjoying life more, being more creative, feeling more connected to nature and other human beings, being more focused at work, and experiencing stress reduction, along with increased energy and vitality.

So what I am truly up to here is helping you live a more satisfying life. Not a bad endgame for any of us, especially in today's challenging times, when we need all the gentle, loving mothers we can get . . . and Mother Nature certainly qualifies! (Except when she turns cold and frosty on you, or pelts you with heavy rain or angry thunder and lightning . . . but even then, you know that in time she will warm up again.)

Now that you know exactly where I am coming from, and how much I want you to at least give these exercises a try, because I do believe they will become addictive—and I mean that in a very positive way!—here are some additional tips to keep you motivated.

• Have a regular buddy to Nancercize with.

• Find or create an outdoor exercise group.

• Schedule a regular time and stick to it until it becomes a habit that's harder to break.

• Usually, it's best to exercise in the morning because so many excuses can come up during the day . . . and it sets the stage for an energized day.

• Find out which type of exercise suits you better—casual or structured—or a combination of both.

• Set goals for yourself or your group and congratulate yourself when you meet them. A good guideline is to increase the intensity or duration by 10% each week, except if you are ill or injured (then you need to cut back for a while).

• Keep track of your progress, using a tracking sheet like this one on page 52, which covers one week: you might want to make copies and put them in a three-hole binder.

• Hire a trainer to work with at least at first to make sure you are doing the exercises correctly.

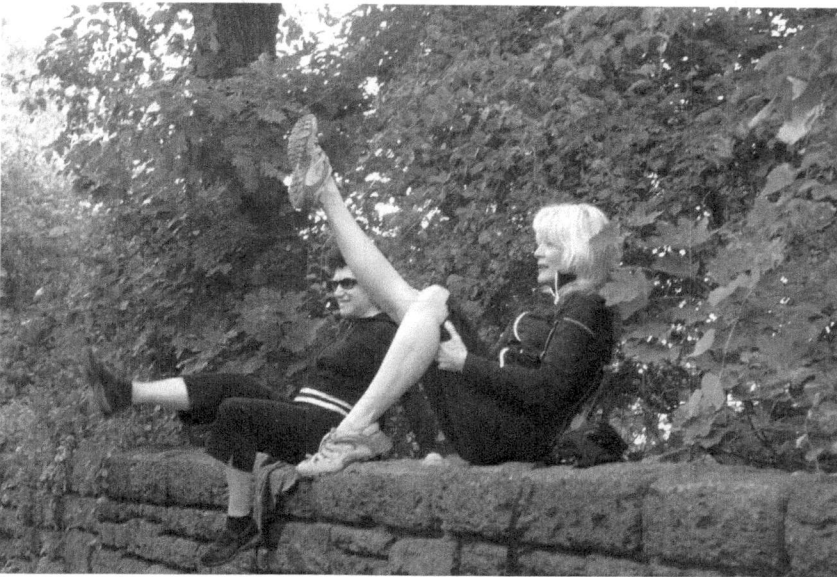

Grab a buddy and Nancercize—on a bench, a wall or wherever your imagination and creativity leads you.

Weekly Nancercize Log

Date	Flexibility	Upper body strength	Lower body strength	Core strength	Endurance	Balance and flexibility

Part II

Stop the 101 Excuses and Do the 101 Exercises
The Exercises and How to Do Them

Flexibility
1. Side stretch
2. Table top stretch
3. Downward facing dog
4. Deep squat stretch
5. Over easy
6. Crossover stretch
7. Hamstring stretch
8. Knee to nose
9. Seated twist
10. Seated eagle
11. Triceps stretch
12. Seated chair pose
13. See-saw
14. Table top twist
15. Flowing lunge
16. Hamstring stretch and twist
17. Crescent stretch
18. Butterfly stretch

19. Upward facing dog
20. Forward flow and twist
21. Wishbone

Lower body strength
22. Hamstring curl
23. Standing donkey side kick
24. Leg circles
25. Hovering squat
26. Stomp on the brake
27. Back leg lift
28. Side leg lift
29. Forward leg lift
30. Static squat
31. Up on your toes
32. Bridge with leg lift
33. Horizon kick
34. L kick
35. Basic squat
36. Squat and cross
37. Tuck and kick
38. Sky kick
39. Xtreme knee lift
40. Split squat
41. Power jump
42. Power taps
43. One-legged squat

Upper body strength
44. Modified push-up
45. Pulsing push-up
46. Push off
47. Walking push-up
48. Push Off and Clap
49. Side plank and arm circle
50. Walk the plank
51. Leg lift push-up

52. Basic dip
53. Cross-legged dip
54. One-legged dip
55. One-arm triceps push-up
56. Power push up
57. One-Armed Power Push-Up
58. Handstand Push-Up
59. Wheelbarrow

Core strength
60. Basic sit-up
61. Hug yourself and twist
62. Hippy dippy plank
63. Basic bicycle
64. Modified plank
65. Double leg lift
66. Scissor kick
67. Flutter kick
68. Roll up
69. Hip lift
70. Elbow plank
71. Knee drop plank
72. Air pump
73. Coasting bicycle
74. Double leg swivel
75. Side sit-up
76. High five sit-up
77. Leg lift plank
78. Thread the Needle

Endurance
79. Slow march
80. Helicopter kick
81. Spider crawl
82. Squat thrust
83. Hooray step-up
84. Tuck jump

CHAPTER ONE

Flexibility

Either you love stretching or you hate it. If you hate it, it's because you don't do it enough or you've been doing it incorrectly! Some people find stretching boring, but more boring to me is to be stiff and have a limited rage of motion in my joints. Although there is controversy over whether stretching actually prevents future injury, there is a logical argument in its favor. If you don't have a full range of motion in a joint, you are likely using the wrong biomechanics to move and, over time, this could lead to tendon problems, tendonitis or tendinopathy, according to the Mayo Clinic.

Plus, when done correctly and regularly, stretching feels really good. Really, really good. And it helps you move more gracefully and youthfully.

Doing stretches on a bench gives you a safe and stable base—like "yoga props" the bench enables you to do the stretch correctly and safely. I've often seen people tense up and struggle to achieve a yoga pose or stretch. That's not relaxing! Benches are like a safety net. Having a bench nearby allows you to find the sweet spot in a stretch—that point of ease and comfort that allows you to relax and feel a stronger, deeper stretch.

You can stretch anytime, anywhere: before exercising, after exercising, in between exercises, or by itself. Just as long as you've warmed up with at least some light aerobics, anything goes except for forcing yourself into a stretch and overdoing it. Stretching shouldn't be scary or uncomfortable or painful. If it is, stop and try something else, or do a gentler version of the stretching move.

Remember, the safest most satisfying and effective way to do a static stretch is to ease into it gradually, breathing slowly and evenly, holding the stretch for up to one minute. I like to make the pose "alive" by working with the breath—release and ease up with the inhale, extend and re-activate with the exhale. Some of the flexibility exercises in this chapter are more "dynamic"—you stretch while moving to increase the range of motion, blood, and oxygen flow to the tissues. These are done with multiple repetitions, and in a flowing manner. Dynamic stretching is usually done before a workout, to warm up the body, while static stretching is most appropriate at the end of a workout when the muscles are already warm and flexible.

1. Side stretch (light)

This stretch is as simple as can be but is a great waker-upper for your side muscles and upper body. In this modification of the "half moon" yoga position, the bench gives you support so you can more comfortably surrender into the movement.

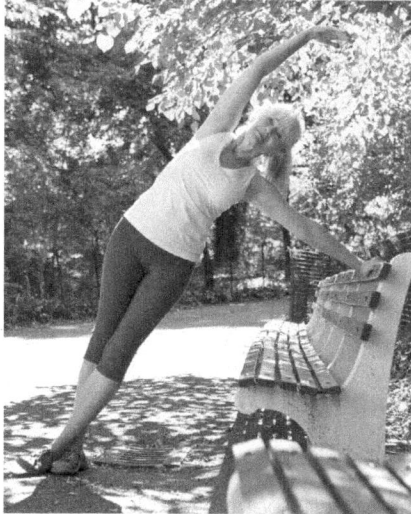

Action

• Stand tall, with your side to the bench, inner hand on the bench back.
• Inhale and reach up and over your body with your free hand.
• Exhale and bend sideways toward the bench from your waist.
• As you inhale and exhale, continue to reach with your free hand, feeling a nice stretch all along your outer side and shoulder.
• Release, and repeat on your other side.

Tips

• Look up at the sky as you keep your shoulders back with your chest open and facing front; don't curl overinwards.
+ Take it up a notch: Place your palm on the bench seat instead of the back, and push your outer hip to the side to get more stretch.
− Tone it down: Place your free hand on your hip instead of reaching overhead.

59

2. Table top stretch (light)

This is a wonderfully simple yet effective stretch for your shoulders, back, hips, and hamstrings. I never leave it out of a workout. Do this anytime and often.

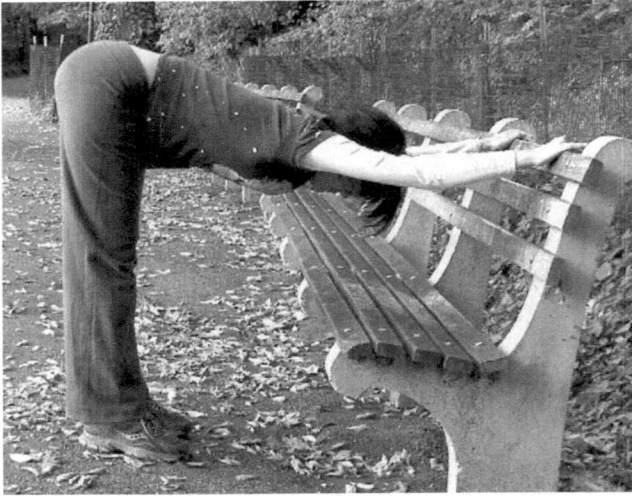

Action
- Stand tall, facing the bench, feet parallel to each other.
- Place both hands on the bench back, shoulder-width apart, as you fold over at the hips, your legs and torso forming a right angle.
- Keeping legs straight and back straight, and heels under your hips, hold for a few inhales and exhales.
- Release, and repeat if you wish.

Tips

- Keep your head and neck in line with your spine.
- Feet can be close together or hip-widthapart. Experiment to see what feels good for you.
- Pull your hips away from the bench, elongating your back.
- **+** Take it up a notch: Press into the bench with your hands and think about bringing your chest to the ground to liven and activate the stretch.
- **–** Tone it down: Bend your knees slightly.

3. Downward facing dog (light)

If you've done yoga, you'll recognize this one. It's a great total body stretch that will also strengthen your upper body and core.

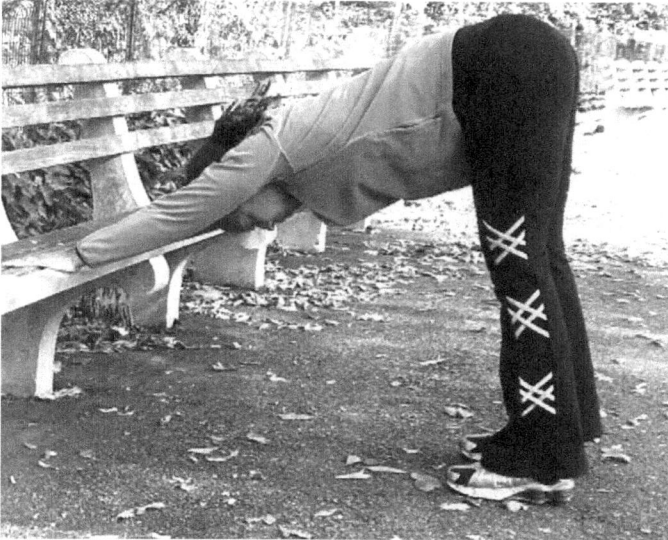

Action
- Stand tall, facing the bench, feet hip-width apart.
- Place both hands on the bench seat, shoulder-width apart, forming a V with your legs and torso.
- Keeping legs straight and back straight, your heels under your hips, hold for a few inhales and exhales.
- Release, and repeat if you wish.

Tips

- Keep your head and neck in line with your spine.
- Pull your hips back and up, away from the bench to stretch them towards the sky.

➕ Take it up a notch: Press into the bench with your hands and think about reaching your chest towards the ground to activate the stretch.

➖ Tone it down: Bend knees slightly if this makes the stretch more comfortable.

61

4. Deep squat stretch (moderate)

I love this stretch after any kind of core work that works the back muscles. But it's also the perfect antidote to too much standing, walking, or sitting.

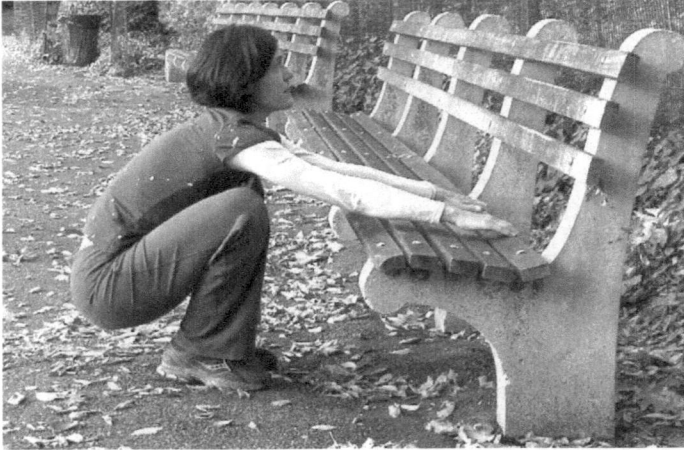

Action

- Stand tall, facing the bench, feet hip-width apart.
- Place both hands on the bench seat, shoulder-width apart, hooking your fingertips over the farthest edge.
- Bend your knees and hips, knees apart and chest between your legs, coming into a squatting position.
- Hold for several inhales and exhales.
- Release, and repeat if you wish.

Tips

- Look straight ahead or keep your head and neck in line with your spine.
- Put most of your bodyweight back in your heels.

➕ Take it up a notch: Pull gently on the seat edge to activate the stretch.

➖ Tone it down: don't go down so far.

5. Over easy (moderate)

This one takes a bit of getting used to, but I love the way gravity helps me stretch the entire back of my body, from head to toe, while the bench supports me. See how long you can chat while in this position!

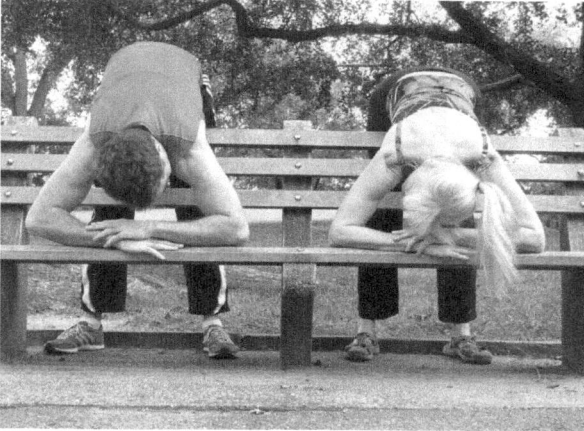

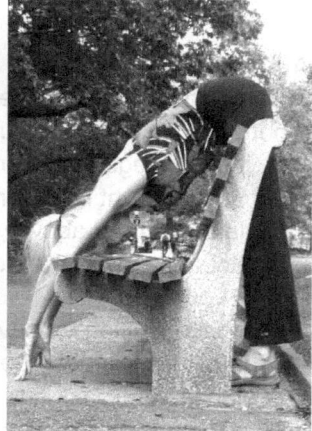

Action

- Facing the back of the bench, place the crease of your hips at the edge of the bench back.
- With hands reaching out in front of you, bend at the hips, draping your torso over the back.
- Allow your forearms to rest on the bench seat, resting your head on your forearms, or not, as your height allows.
- Inhale and exhale as you allow gravity to stretch your back and shoulders.
- Release, and repeat if you wish.

Tips

➕ Take it up a notch: Stretch out your arms and place your fingertips on the ground.

6. Crossover stretch (moderate)

Your hips and knees will thank you for doing the crossover. This position improves your ability to move your hips, and helps re-align your pelvis. So, maybe that special someone will thank you too.

Action

- Sit tall on the edge of the bench, both feet flat on the ground in front of you with legs at a right angle.
- Cross your right leg over your left, ankle resting just above your knee.
- Gently and slowly lean forward from your hips.
- Hold this position for several inhales and exhales, feeling the stretch in your back and hips.
- Slowly bring your torso back to upright and repeat with the other leg.

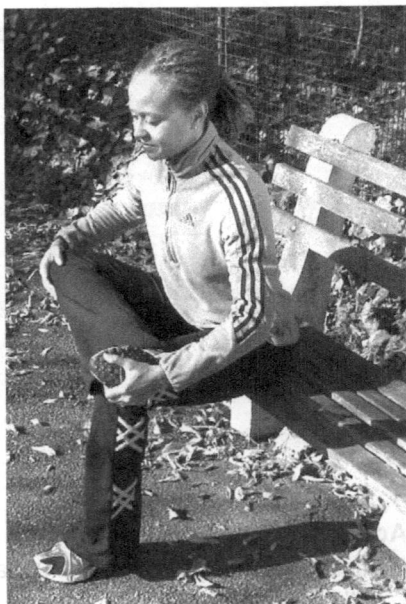

Tips

- Sit at the edge of the bench, rather than towards the back.
- Feel elongated in your torso as you fold, keep your back relatively straight, rather than curved, head in line with your spine. The idea is not to see how far down your head can go; instead, you are trying to reach out with your chest.!
- You may be more comfortable if the bench has a flat seat, rather than a curved one.
- ➕ Take it up a notch: Press your crossed leg down into the support leg to activate the stretch.
- ➖ Tone it down: support your knees in the palm of your hand.

7. Flowing hamstring stretch (intense)

Work up to doing this two-part stretch a dozen times on each side with coordinated breathing to get into the flow!

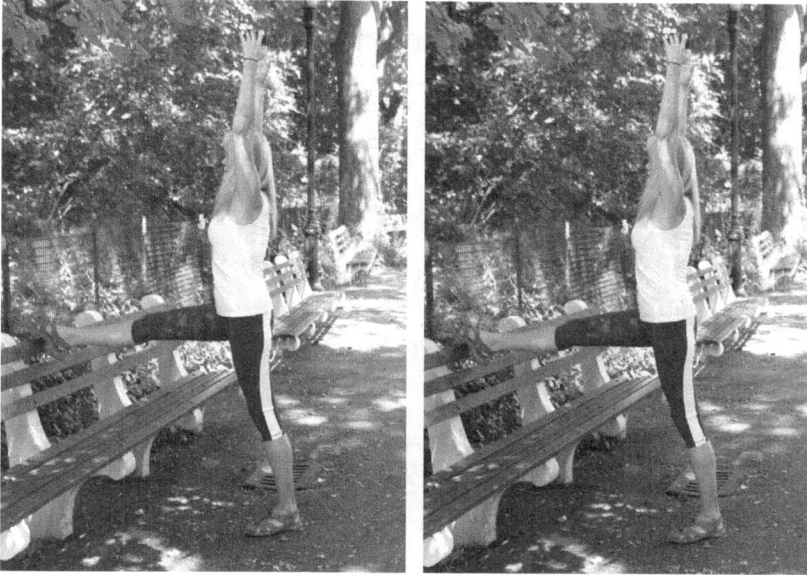

Action
- Stand tall, facing the bench.
- Place your foot on the back of the bench.
- Inhale and raise both arms over your heard, elongating your torso.
- Exhale and lean forward and fold over at your hips, hands resting wherever is comfortable—your shin, foot, or the back of the bench.
- Hold for several inhales and exhales.
- Slowly return your torso to upright and repeat with your other leg.

Tips

- Try to keep your back as straight as possible, head in line with your spine, even if that means you don't touch your toes!
- Avoid locking your knees—keep the knees slightly soft.
- ✚ Take it up a notch: Pull slightly on the bench back to activate the stretch.
- ▬ Tone it down: Place your foot on the bench seat rather than the back.

65

8. Knee to nose (moderate)

So simple yet so blissful— you'd think it would be against the law! This set of stretches works on your hips, back, and shoulders. Confession: I often do this plus a twist in the morning before getting out of bed!

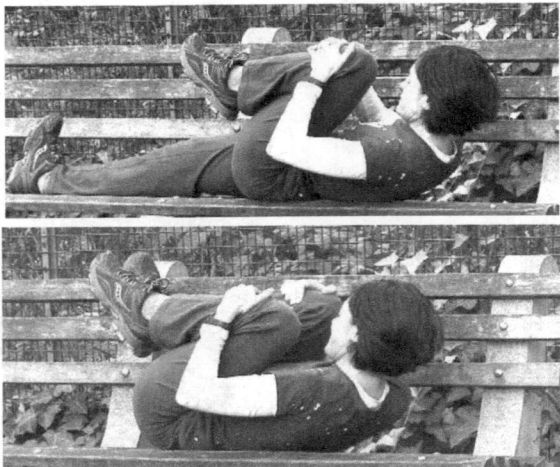

Action
- Lie on the bench seat with your legs extended.
- As you lift your head, bring your left knee towards your nose or forehead, gently clasping your hands around your knee for extra stretch.
- Hold this position for a few inhales and exhales.
- Return your leg and head to starting position and repeat with the other leg.
- To complete the stretch, gently hug both your knees to your chest and hold for a few inhales and exhales.

Tips

- If you have any knee issues, place your hands under your knees, on the back of your upper thigh, rather than on top of your knees.
- You may be most comfortable on a bench that has a flat, rather than rounded seat, or one that has no back.

➕ Take it up a notch: Press your legs gently into your hands to activate the stretch.

➖ Tone it down: Leave your head down on the bench during the stretches.

66

9. Seated twist (light)

We seldom realize how little mobility we have in our spines until we twist suddenly and hurt ourselves! Do this gentle twist regularly to keep your spine and neck nimble and graceful.

Action
- Sit tall on the bench, all the way back, close to the bench back, your feet parallel and hip-width apart.
- Twist to one side placing one hand on your outer thigh and the other on the bench back.
- Hold this position for a few inhales and exhales, deepening the twist with each exhale.
- Slowly unwind and twist to the other side.

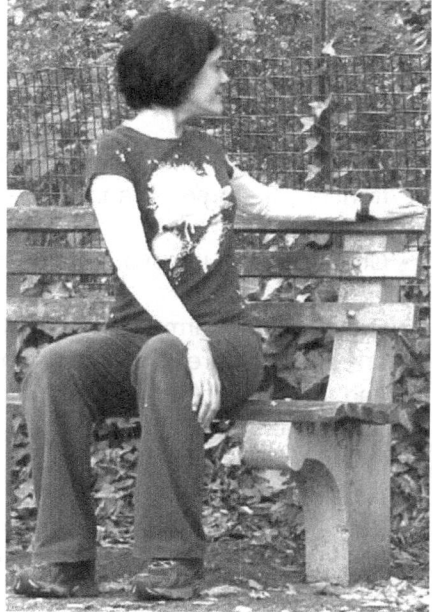

Tips

- Keep your shoulders relaxed and even, rather than allowing them to shrug up towards your ears.
- Make sure your head follows the direction of the twist, to give your neck muscles a nice stretch as well.

➕ Take it up a notch: Press gently against your thigh and pull slightly on the bench back to activate the stretch. As you inhale, draw your belly towards your spine and deepen the stretch.

➖ Tone it down: place your hand on the bench seat rather than the back.

10. Seated eagle (moderate)

A classic standing yoga pose that stretches shoulders and hips and challenges your balance, the eagle is a toughie for many people. Doing it while seated on a park bench puts it within reach so you get the benefits without falling down and feeling like anything but a noble eagle. Once you have your confidence, you can try it standing

Action
- Sit on the edge of the bench, feet in front of you, torso tall and elongated.
- Cross your left leg over your right leg.
- Cross your left arm over your right arm, so your forearms are upright and the backs of your hands touch each other.
- Hold for several inhales and exhales.
- Slowly release and repeat on the other side, reversing the positions of your arms and legs.

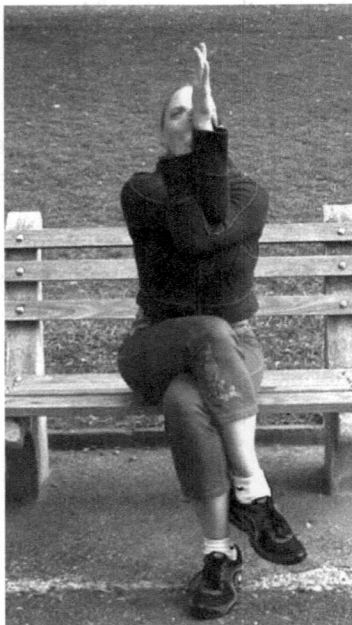

Tips

- Keep your shoulders relaxed and even, rather than shrugging the mallowing them to shrug up towards your ears.
- **+** Take it up a notch: Try hooking one foot behind the ankle of your other foot, and one hand around the other hand, palms touching.
- **−** Tone it down: Do just the arms or just the legs.

11. Triceps stretch (light)

This is the perfect stretch after doing dips or push-ups, but you'll also find stretching the back of your arms (triceps muscles) and shoulders to be relaxing any time.

Action
- Sit on the bench with your torso elongated.
- Reach up with one arm, bend it at the elbow so your forearm is behind your head. Your hand should fall between your shoulder blades on your back.
- Grab the elbow with your other hand and gently press so the back of your arm feels the stretch.
- Hold the position for a few inhales and exhales.
- Release, and repeat with the other side.

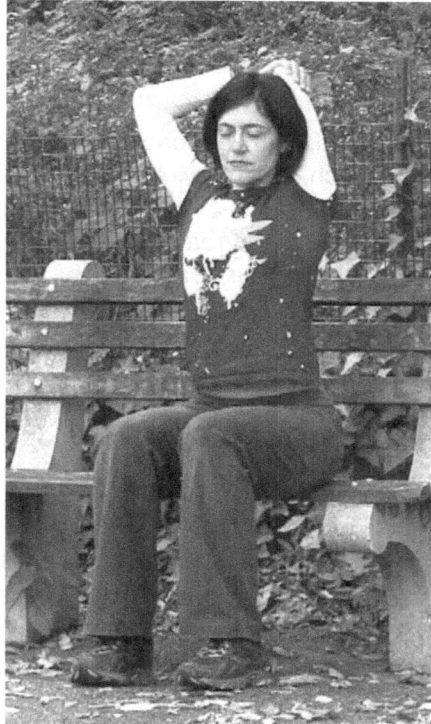

Tips

• Try not to let your head and chin jut forward.

➕ Take it up a notch: Let your stretching arm press back slightly against your hand, giving it resistance and activating the stretch.

➖ Tone it down: Omit grabbing the elbow with the other hand.

69

12. Seated chair pose (light)

Another challenging yoga pose when done standing, made more do-able for more people by adding a bench. This gentle stretch elongates your torso and opens up your shoulder

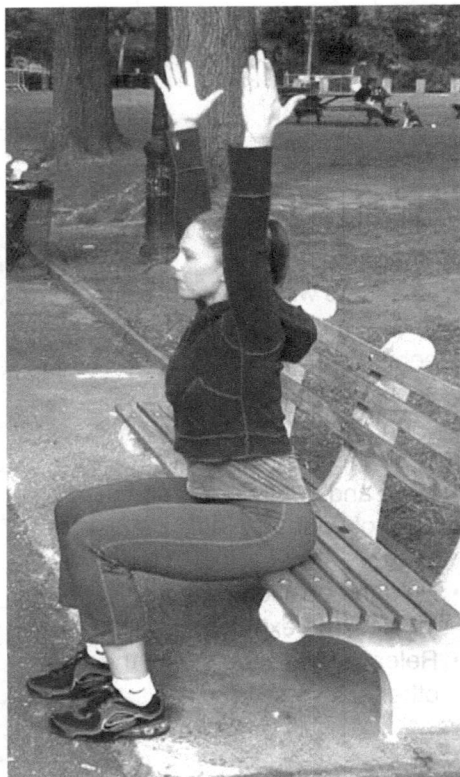

Action
- Stand tall, with your back to the bench, feet parallel and hip-width apart.
- Slowly raise and reach your arms above your head.
- Slowly sit on the edge of the bench.
- Hold this position for a few inhales and exhales.
- Release, and repeat if you wish.

Tips

• Keep your shoulders relaxed and even, rather than allowing them to shrug up towards your ears.

➕ Take it up a notch: Try standing up with your bottom a few inches away from the bench and holding it for a few breaths. This will activate the stretch and make it more intense.

➖ Tone it down: Bend your elbows and intertwine your fingers behind your head instead of holding them up vertically.

13. See-saw (intense)

This requires a partner and is so much fun you won't even realize what great things are happening to your back, shoulders, hips and arms. Along with the swings and the monkey bars, I always looked forward to playing on the seesaws in the playground of my youth. Go on, grab a playmate and enjoy your second childhood.

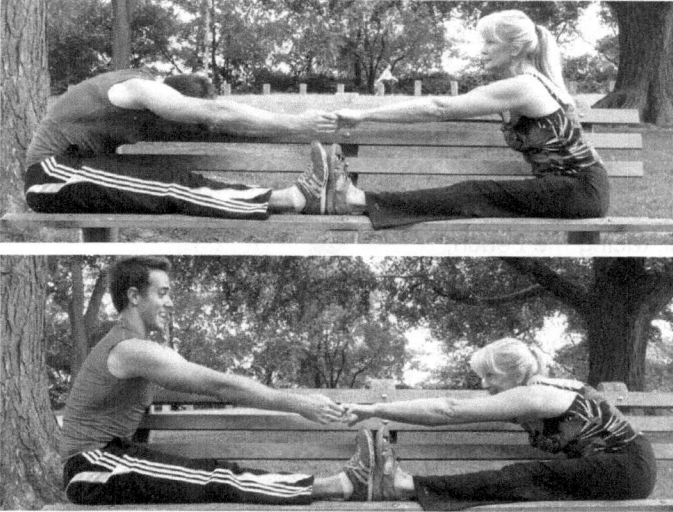

Action
- Grab a partner.
- Both of you sit on the bench, with legs straight, soles of your feet touching.
- Sit up straight and clasp each other's hands..
- As one of you folds forward at hips, the other pulls gently and leans back.
- Hold for a few inhales and exhales.
- Reverse positions slowly.

Tips

- This is most comfortable on a bench with a flat seat rather than a curved one. You also might prefer a bench with no back.
- Keep your head in line with your spine. (If your exercise partner is as attractive as mine, admittedly, this will be difficult.)
- — Tone it down: Keep your knees slightly bent.

14. Table top twist (light)

I will often combine this with the table top stretch (#2), hence the name. One flows perfectly into the other, giving your spine a complete treat.

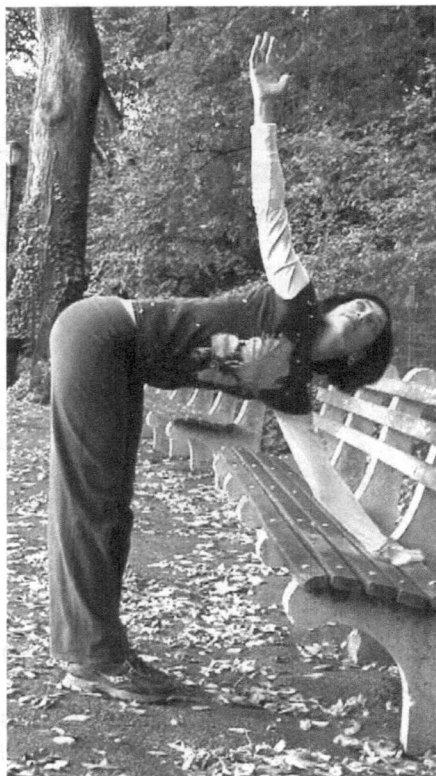

Action
- Stand tall, facing the bench, feet parallel to each other.
- Lean over, bending at your hips and resting your hands on the bench seat.
- Sweep one arm out to the side and up, looking up toward the sky and twisting.
- Hold for a few inhales and exhales.
- Sweep your arm down and repeat on the other side.

Tips

• Keep your legs straight, but knees not locked, feet flat on the ground.

➕ Take it up a notch: Twist more deeply, aiming to bring your shoulder back and your chest towards the sky.

➖ Tone it down: Rest your free hand on the bench back and twist gently while gazing straight ahead or down.

15. Flowing lunge (moderate)

This series is part of a longer sequence of flowing yoga poses called the Sun Salutation. The bench supports you in an easier position than the classic hands-on-floor position, and repeating the exercises several times warms up and stretches your hips, back, legs, and shoulders. Be careful not to bump your knee on the bench when you step forward into the lunge!

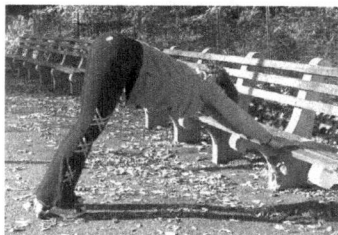

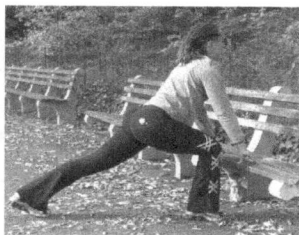

Action
- Stand tall, facing the bench, feet hip-width apart.
- Place both hands on the bench seat, shoulder-width apart, your feet under your hips, forming an upside down V shape with your legs and torso.
- Pull your hips back away from the bench, elongating your spine and torso.
- Bend one leg and take a step forward, placing our foot directly under your hands, in a lunge position.
- Release the foot back to return to the starting upside down V position and repeat, taking a step with the other leg.

Tips

- Keep your head and neck on a line with your spine.
- Be sure your knee is directly over your ankle in the lunge position, not past it.
- Be careful not to bump your knee on the bench when you step forward into the lunge!

➕ Take it up a notch: Press into the bench with your hands as you think about reaching your chest to the ground to activate the first part of the stretch.

➖ Tone it down: Try this from the rear of the bench, and use the bench back rather than the bench seat to support you as you lunge forward.

16. Hamstring stretch and twist (light)

Here's a nice gentle little twist that opens up your spine, neck, shoulders, and back of your legs. Do it anytime!

Action
- Stand tall, facing the bench, feet parallel to each other.
- Lift one leg, resting the heel on the seat of the bench,
- Twist your torso towards the lifted leg and place your oppsite hand on the outside of your leg, other hand on hip or waist.
- Hold for a few inhales and exhales.
- Release and repeat on the other side.

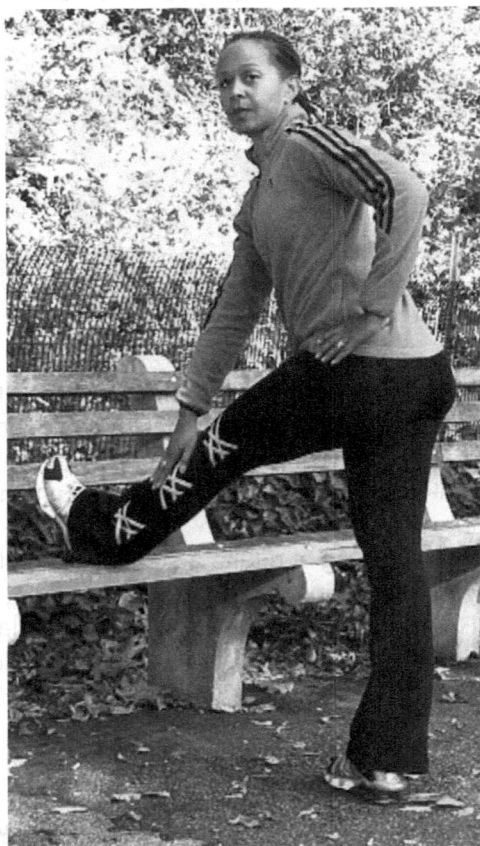

Tips

- Keep your legs straight, but do not lock your knees; rather, keep them slightly soft.
- ➕ Take it up a notch: Place your heel on the bench back.
- ➖ Tone it down: Just put your foot forward under the bench on the ground.

17. Crescent stretch (intense)

This yoga stretch looks as glorious as it feels. Enjoy how your entire body expands and opens up.

Action
- Stand with your side to the bench.
- Tilt your torso towards the bench, allowing your inside hand to rest on the seat.
- Reach up with your outside hand, while crossing the inside leg in front.
- Look up, forming a crescent shape with your body.
- Hold for several inhales and exhales.
- Release and repeat on the other side.

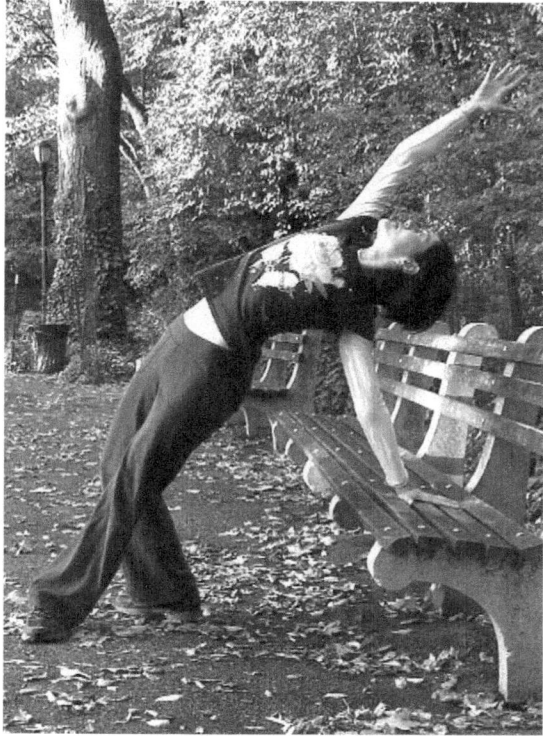

Tips

- Slightly bend your legs in synch with your breaths to get more stretch and enliven the position.
- Keep your shoulders down, rather than jammed up around your ears.
- Remember to smile!
- Take it down a notch: Place your hand on the back of the bench rather than the seat.

18. Butterfly stretch (intense)

There is no finer groin stretcher around! This will also help increase your flexibility in your hips and lower back, while simultaneously stretching the muscles of your inner thighs.

Action
- Sit tall on the bench and bring your heels as close to your pelvis as is comfortable.
- Grasp your ankles, toes, or shins while keeping your back elongated and straight, allowing your knees to drop down as far as they will go comfortably go.
- Hold this position for a few inhales and exhales, growing taller with each inhale.

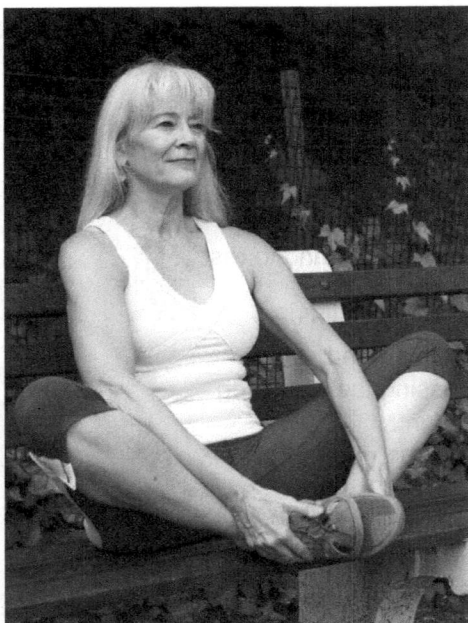

Tips

- Look straight ahead, with your head aligned with your spine.
- Avoid forcing your knees to go down; rather, think of releasing the tops of your thighbones towards the bench.

➕ Take it up a notch: Lean forward with a straight back, keeping your abs in and your shoulders down and as you press your knees down more.

➖ Tone it down: Leave one foot on the ground, and bring up one leg at a time, resting the sole of your foot on the inside of your other thigh. This also helps if you feel discomfort in your knees while doing the full butterfly.

76

19. Upward facing dog (moderate)

This yoga pose stretches your chest, shoulders, and abdomen while it strengthens your arms and improves posture. It's often part of the flowing Sun Salutation sequence but can be done individually as well.

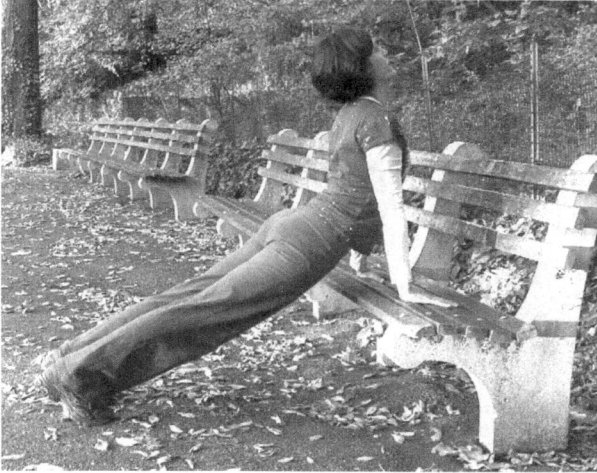

Action

- Stand tall, facing the bench.
- Place both palms on the bench seat, shoulder-width apart, arms perpendicular to the ground.
- Step your feet back away from the bench, with your toes on the ground hip-width apart.
- Lean your chest forward, holding your weight on your arms, forming a slight arch in your back.
- Hold for a few inhales and exhales.
- Release, and repeat if you wish.

Tips

• Keep your shoulders down, away from your ears.
• Arms and legs are straight, but avoid locking your knees or elbows.
➕ Take it up a notch: Tilt your head back and look up to the sky to increase the backbend in this stretch.
➖ Tone it down: Place your hands on the back of the bench instead of the seat.

77

20. Forward flow and twist (intense)

This flowing sequence stretches and elongates the whole back of your body—shoulders, back, and legs—while limbering up your spine.

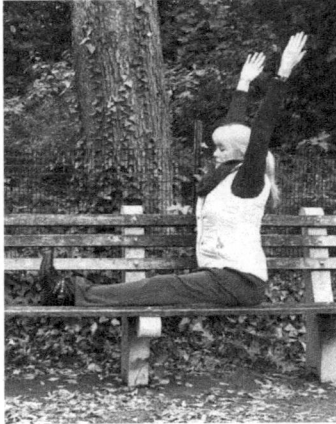

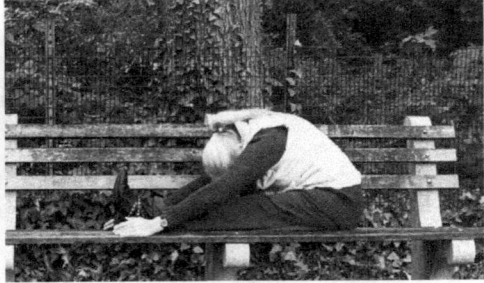

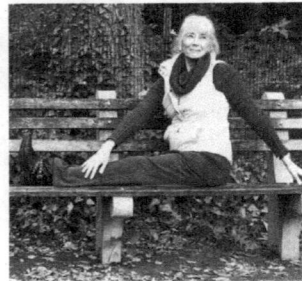

Action

- Sit tall on the bench with your legs together, stretched out before you. Inhale, elongating your torso further and raising your arms overhead.
- Exhale and fold forward from your hips, allowing your hands to fall on the bench outside your legs.
- Hold for a few inhales and exhales, releasing slightly with the inhale and going deeper into the stretch with your exhale. Inhaling, raise your torso, arms overhead.
- Exhale as you lower your arms, twisting to one side, allowing your hands to rest on the bench.
- Repeat the sequence, twisting to the other side.

Tips

- Keep your torso and neck elongated throughout.
- This will be most comfortable on a bench with a flat, rather than curved seat. You might also prefer a bench without a back.
- ➕ Take it up a notch: reach past your feet and interlace your fingers.
- ➖ Tone it down: Bend your knees slightly and as you bend forward.

21. Wishbone (intense)

I remember the first time I did this standing up in a yoga class—it was thrilling! There's a famous video of the musician and composer Sting practicing this and other yoga positions before giving a concert. Impressive!

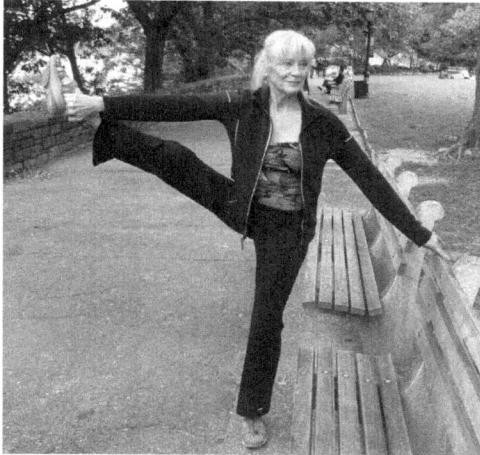

Action

- Stand with your side to the bench. Place your inside hand on the bench back.
- Bend your outside leg and grab your heel, toes or instep from the inside with your free outside hand.
- Gradually straighten your leg.
- Hold for several inhales and exhales.
- Release, and repeat on the other side.

Tips

- Keep your knees soft—avoid locking your knees.
- To activate the stretch, slightly bend your outside leg with each inhale and straighten with each exhale.

➕ Take it up a notch: Gradually lift your leg higher and higher. Then let go of the bench!

➖ Tone it down: Grab the inside of your calf rather than your foot. You can also try this stretch with your leg resting on the bench seat or back, rather than holding it up by yourself in the air with your hand.

CHAPTER TWO

Lower Body Strength

It always distresses me to learn when someone is ignoring their strengthening exercises. I can understand not liking weights or machines in a health club, or exercise bands, but that's why Nancercize strengthening exercises use just your own bodyweight. You don't need any equipment to tone and strengthen your muscles.

Strong muscles not only feel great, they look great and help you move more powerfully and gracefully. Your clothes will fit better, and because muscles improve your metabolism, building up your lower body will help you lose fat, inches, and weight more easily . . . and help you keep it off. That's because "muscle dictates metabolism"—you need to build muscle to boost your body's ability to burn calories even hours after you've finished exercising.

Strengthening exercises are also the best way to counteract the muscle shrinkage and bone thinning that happens to us, as we get older . . . we lose muscle and bone where we need it, and gain fat where we don't . . . unless we build muscle and bone through resistance exercise.

In this section, I give you about two dozen ways to sculpt your lower body—your legs, hips, and derrière. If you're short on time—and who isn't?—gravitate toward those exercises that also tend to work the core at the same time.

Remember to train each major muscle group in your lower body two or three days each week, using a variety of exercises. You should wait at least 48 hours between resistance training exercises of a particular muscle group. So, for example, if you work your legs hard on Tuesday, wait until Thursday to target them again. Remember, choose light intensity exercises if you are older or a previously sedentary adult just starting to exercise, or starting to do resistance training for the first time (or for the first time in a long time).

The current recommendations are that you do 8-12 repetitions to improve strength and power, 10-15 repetitions to improve strength in middle-age and older persons starting exercise, and 15-20 repetitions to improve muscular endurance. Or, if you're not the type who likes to keep track, there's a simpler way. Just repeat each exercise until you can't do any more ("muscle failure"), and move on and move on to the next exercise. You can do one "set" of repetitions, rest for a minute or so, and then do another set or two.

22. Hamstring curl (moderate)

Hamstring curls will give you a nice toned curve on the backs of your thighs, and work the front of your thighs and your gluteus muscles as well.

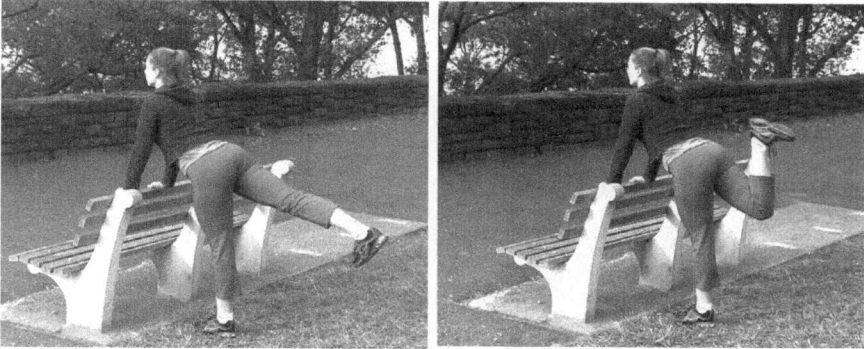

Action
- Stand tall behind the bench, feet together.
- Place both hands on the bench back.
- Leaning forward slightly, raise one leg behind you until it's at the same height as your hip.
- Keeping the leg up there, bend the knee of the raised leg, bringing your heel towards your buttocks.
- Straighten your leg, extending it out long behind you.
- Repeat as many times as you can.
- Repeat with your other leg.

Tips

- Keep your neck long, your arms and back straight and long and your gaze straight ahead.
- Keep your body even, with both your hips on the same plane.
- Don't move your knee during this exercise, just your calf.
- You may be most comfortable using a bench with a rounded edge.
- ✚ Take it up a notch: Let go of the bench while you bend and straighten your leg, arms out to your side (or in front of you) for balance. This will also work your core muscles.
- ― Tone it down: Keep your leg lower than hip level.

83

23. Standing donkey side kick (moderate)

This is one of a variety of kicks that will give you nice, round, firm buttocks. The bench offers a comfortable alternative to doing the kicks on all fours on the floor, which can be rough on your wrists and knees.

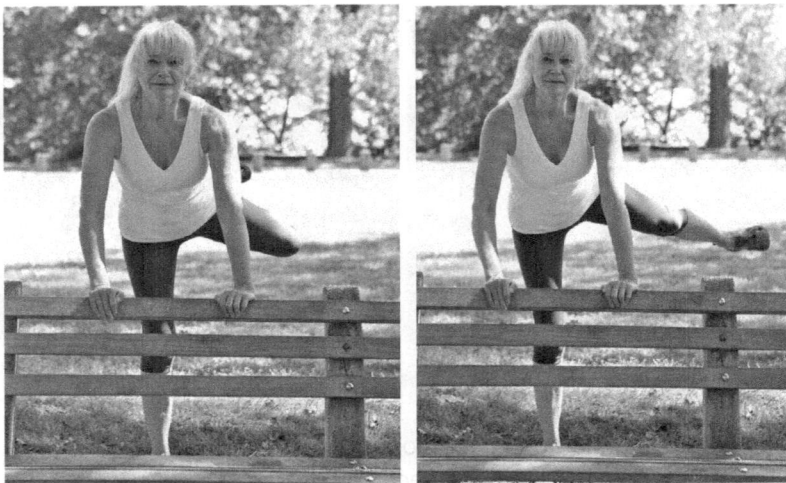

Action
• Stand tall behind the bench, feet together, and place both hands on the bench back.
• Bend the knee of one leg as you raise it out to the side, about as high as your hip.
• Straighten the leg, extending it out long to the side.
• Keeping the leg at hip height, bend the knee so your heel comes towards your buttocks.
• Repeat as many times as you can.
• Repeat with your other leg.

Tips

• Keep your neck long, your arms and back straight and long and your gaze straight ahead.
• Keep your body even, with both your hips on the same plane.
➕ Take it up a notch: Let go of the bench while you bend and straighten your leg, arms out to your sides (or in front of you) for balance; this will also work your core muscles.

24. Leg circles (moderate)

Leg circles hit all the hip and gluteus muscles and lead to a firm, rounded derrière. You don't need to make big circles—they just need to be round. No square circles!

Action

- Stand tall behind the bench, feet together; place both hands on the bench back.
- Raise one leg behind you until it's at about hip height.
- Keeping the leg extended out long behind you, draw a circle in the air with your foot, making circles with the entire leg.
- Make at least 10 circles, and then reverse the direction for 10 more circles.
- Repeat with your other leg.

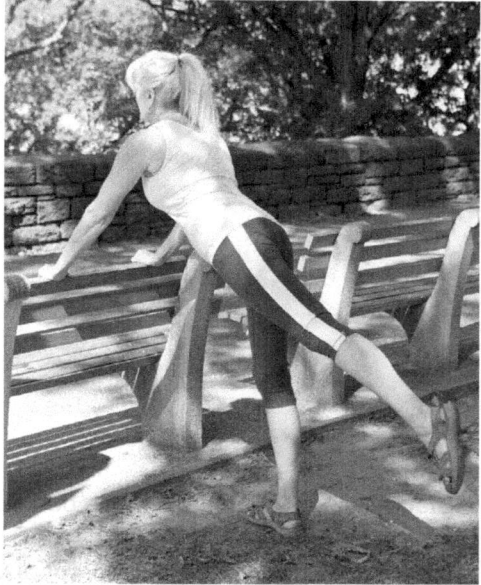

Tips

- Keep your neck long, your arms and back straight and long and your gaze straight ahead.
- Keep your body even, with both your hips on the same plane.
- You may be most comfortable using a bench with a rounded edge.
- ✚ Take it up a notch: Let go of the bench while you draw the circle, arms out to your sides (or in front of you) for balance; this works your core muscles as well.

25. Hovering squat (moderate)

Squats are one of the very best all-round things you can do for your thighs, hips, and buttocks. Often, people either don't squat low enough for it to be effective, or they squat too low, jeopardizing the future life of their knees. This version sets you up for doing squats using the best form for most people.

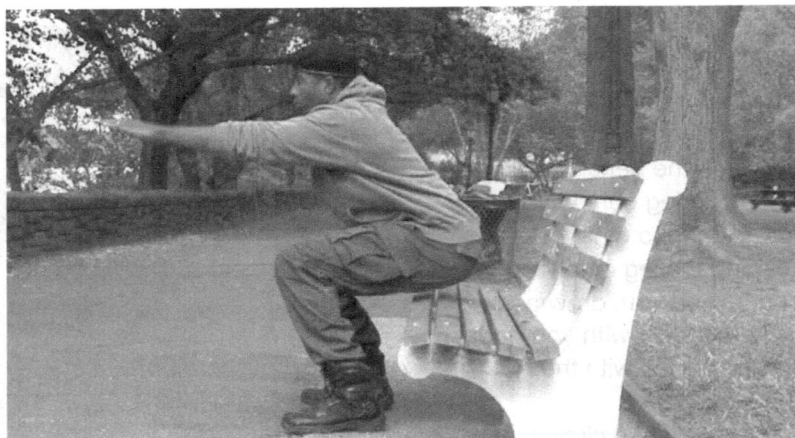

Action
- Stand tall, with your back to the bench, feet parallel and hip-width apart.
- Raise and reach your arms in front of you, about shoulder level.
- Slowly lower your hips towards the seat of the bench, but stop just short of sitting all the way down.
- Hold this position for a few inhales and exhales (20-30 seconds); then stand up.
- Repeat as many times as you can.

Tips

- Keep your shoulders relaxed and even, rather than allowing them to shrug up towards your ears.
- Put most of your bodyweight back in your heels.
- Don't let your knees extend forward past your toes.

➕ Take it up a notch: Pulse your body up and down an inch or two in the squatting position.

➖ Tone it down: Don't go down so far, or don't hold the pose as long.

26. Stomp on the brake (moderate)

Often we work our legs and hips to the front only, shortchanging the muscles to the side. When you stomp on the brake you're engaging many more muscles, improving your strength and flexibility while engaging your core muscles.

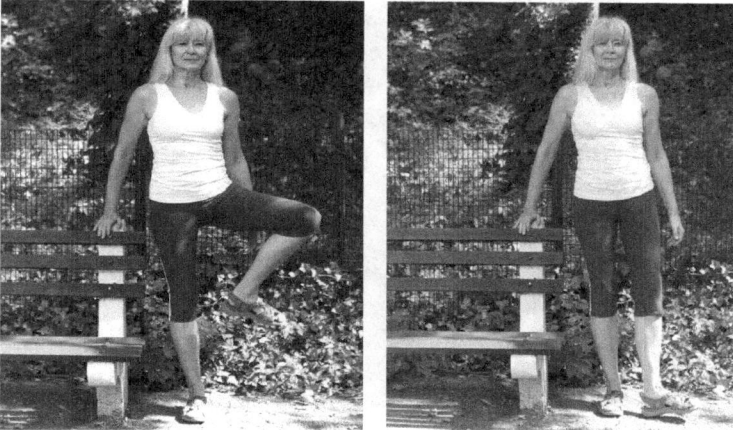

Action

- Stand tall beside the bench, feet together, placing your inside hand on the bench back for support.
- Bend your outside knee up towards your shoulder as high as you can while still standing up straight; then turn it out.
- Keeping your knee turned out, press down with your foot as if you were stepping on a brake, without touching the ground.
- Repeat, raising your knee and pressing down with your foot as many times as you can, in a pumping action.
- Repeat with your other leg.

Tips

- Keep your neck long, your back straight and long and your gaze straight ahead.
- Try not to lean to the side in order to raise your leg higher—that's cheating!

➕ Take it up a notch: Let go of the bench while you pump, arms out to each side for balance.

➖ Tone it down: Raise your leg just a few inches off the ground.

87

27. Back leg lift (light)

This simple move works the back of your legs, hips, and backside. Just remember to squeeze those muscles and keep the working leg off the ground the entire time!

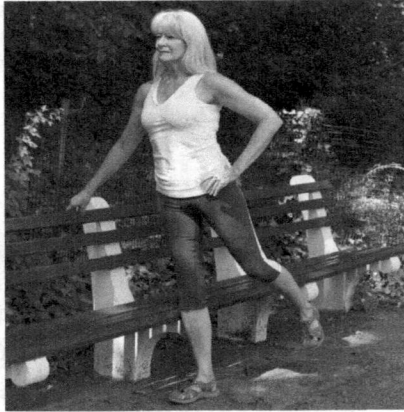

Action
- Stand tall with your side to the bench, feet together.
- Place your inside hand on the bench back and your outside hand on your hip.
- Bring your outside leg up behind you as high as you can while still standing up straight.
- Lower the leg, without touching the ground.
- Repeat raising and lowering your leg as many times as you can.
- Switch sides and repeat with your other leg.

Tips

- Keep your neck long, your back straight and long and your gaze straight ahead.
- Try not to lean forward in order to raise your leg higher—that's cheating!

➕ Take it up a notch: Let go of the bench while you raise and lower your leg, arms out to your side (or in front of you) for balance; this will engage your core muscles more as well.

➖ Tone it down: Raise your leg just a few inches off the ground.

28. Side leg lift (light)

We rarely move our legs to the side during everyday activities. This exercise corrects the tendency to move our limbs in the forward-backward plane exclusively and gets those side muscles working.

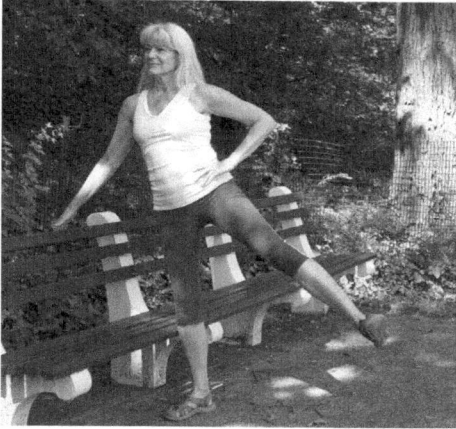

Action
- Stand tall with your side towards the bench, feet together.
- Place your inside hand on the bench back and your outside hand on your hip.
- Bring your outside leg up and out to the side as high as you can while still standing up straight.
- Lower the leg, preferably without touching the ground.
- Repeat raising and lowering your leg as many times as you can.
- Switch sides and repeat with your other leg.

Tips

- Keep your neck long, your back straight and long and your gaze straight ahead.
- Try not to lean to the side in order to raise your leg higher—that's cheating!

+ Take it up a notch: Let go of the bench while you raise and lower your leg, arms out to your side for balance.

− Tone it down: Raise your leg just a few inches off the ground.

29. Forward leg lift (light)

This leg lift works not only your thigh and hip muscles, but your core muscles as well. The challenge with this deceptively simple exercise is to engage your core muscles to keep your torso vertical, rather than leaning back.

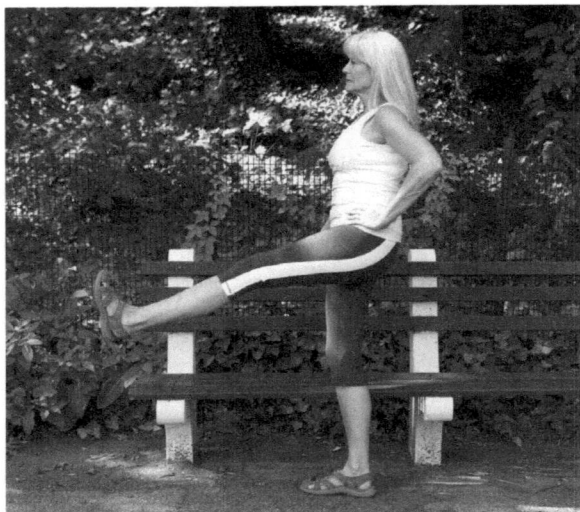

Action
- Stand tall with your side towards the bench, feet together.
- Place your inside hand on the bench back and your outside hand on your hip.
- Bring your outside leg up in front of you as high as you can while still standing up straight.
- Lower the leg, preferably without touching the ground.
- Repeat raising and lowering your leg as many times as you can.
- Switch sides and repeat with your other leg.

Tips

- Keep your neck long, your back straight and long and your gaze straight ahead.
- Try not to lean backward in order to raise your leg higher—that's cheating!
- Take it up a notch: Let go of the bench while you raise and lower your leg, arms out to your side (or in front of you) for balance.
- Tone it down: Raise your leg just a few inches off the ground.

90

30. Static squat (moderate)

Squats are the go-to exercise for working your butt, hips, and legs. But did you know that when you squat you're also working your core muscles, toning your midsection? You might find this variation to be easier on your knees; a plus is that it also works the arms and shoulders.

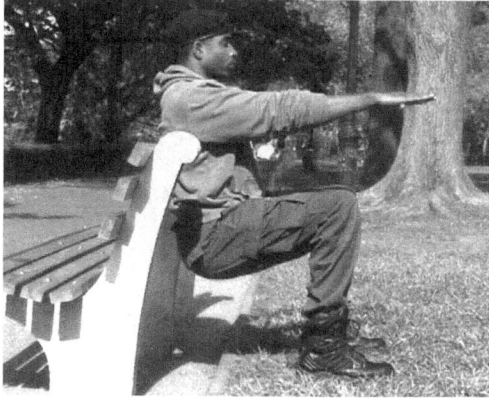

Action
- Stand tall, behind the bench, facing away from it, feet about hip-width apart and 2 feet away from the bench
- Reach behind you and rest your palms on the top edge, while bending your knees and leaning against the bench back.
- Keep bending your knees as your body slides down the bench back until your thighs are parallel with the ground.
- Let your hands swing forward in front of you, while pressing your lower back into the bench.
- Hold for as long as you can (up to one minute and at least 10-30 seconds).

Tips

- Keep your neck long, your back straight and long and your gaze straight ahead.
- Keep your weight in your heels and your knees over your ankles.
- ➕ Take it up a notch: Lower your body closer to the ground unless it bothers your knees.
- ➖ Tone it down: Lower your body less.

31. Up on your toes (light)

Calf raises are the classic way to strengthen your feet and ankles and to develop your calves. I'm pretty sure this is how Baryshnikov started.

Action
- Stand tall, facing the back of the bench, feet parallel and a few inches apart. (Unless you're really tall and need to bend over a bit.)
- Rest both hands on the bench back for support.
- Rise up on your toes and then lower back down.
- Do as many calf raises as you can.
- Repeat with your toes pointing outward, heels together.
- Repeat with your heels pointing outward, toes together.

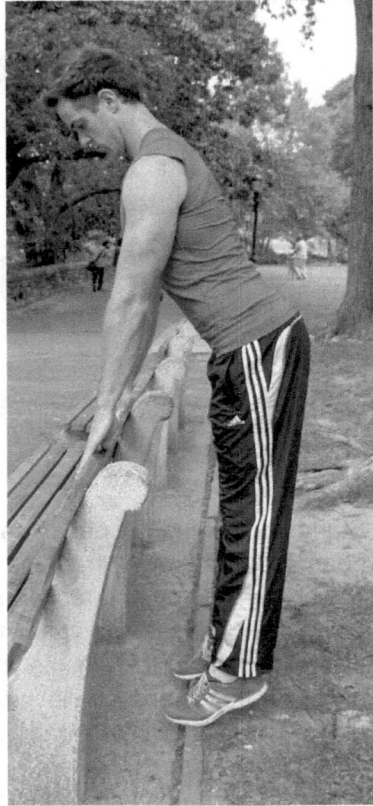

Tips

- Gradually start to do your calf raises without the bench or other support, to improve your balance as well.
- Once you can do these without support, you can sneak them in anywhere—while waiting for the elevator, or the bus or subway, or any time you find yourself bored while standing.

➕ Take it up a notch: Do these balancing on one foot at a time. Or, do them on a step or curb, so your heel drops down below the standing position before you rise up on your toes.

➖ Tone it down: do these while seated on the bench.

92

32. Bridge with leg lift (moderate)

This bridge variation really isolates the gluteus (butt) muscles and the hamstrings of the back of your thighs. Done correctly, it will also work your core muscles.

Action

- Lie face up on the bench seat, knees bent, feet flat on the bench, and hands by your sides.
- Contract your butt, hamstring, and abdominal muscles and curl your hips and torso up, supporting your weight on your feet, shoulders, and arms. Your hands may grip the edge of the bench on each side for leverage.
- Straighten one leg up, heel flexed, keeping your back in one straight line (no sagging!)
- Hold for as long as possible (at least 10-30 seconds) before curling down.
- Repeat with your other leg.

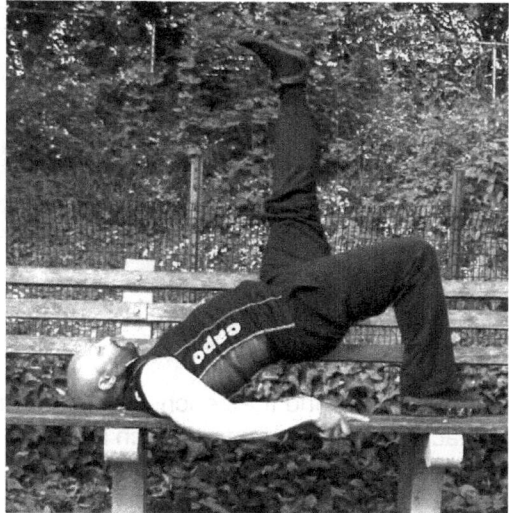

Tips

- Make sure you contract your gluteus, abs, and hamstrings to raise the hips, rather than just driving your supporting foot downward and hyperextending your lower back.
- This works best on a flat bench with no back.
- ➕ Take it up a notch: Pulse your hips up and down one inch while you hold the position.
- ➖ Tone it down. Do the bridge keeping both feet on the bench, without raising your leg.

93

33. Horizon kick (intense)

This is another deceptively simple move that works more of your body than the butt and hips that meet the eye. Your standing leg, for example, will be talking back to you—and your core will be thanking you.

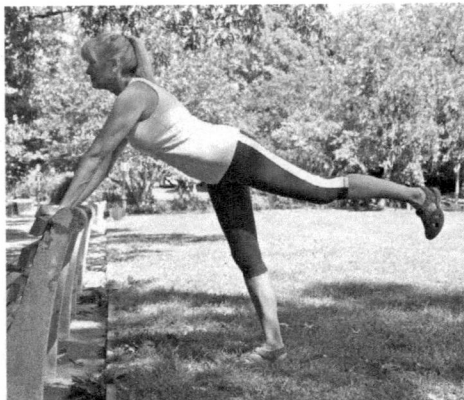

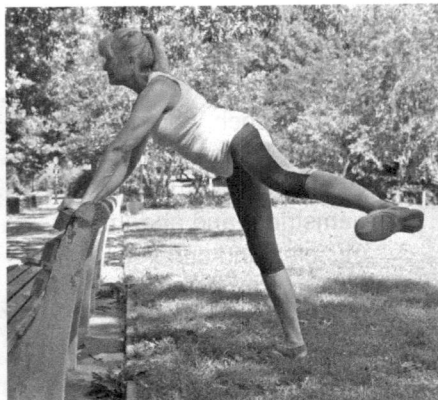

Action
- Stand tall behind the bench, feet together.
- Place both hands on the bench back.
- Raise one leg behind you, about as high as your hip.
- Kick the leg to the side slowly, towards your shoulder and the bench.
- Kick it back to starting position and repeat as many times as you can.
- Repeat with your other leg.

Tips

- Keep your neck long, your arms and back straight and long and your gaze straight ahead.
- Keep your body even, with both your hips on the same plane.
- You may be most comfortable using a bench with a rounded edge.
- ➕ Take it up a notch: Let go of the bench while you do the kicks, arms out to your side (or in front of you) for balance.
- ➖ Tone it down: Kick with your leg lower to the ground.

94

34. L-kick (moderate)

Don't be deceived by the casual, seemingly relaxed position. This kick is amazingly effective for hips, thighs, and core.

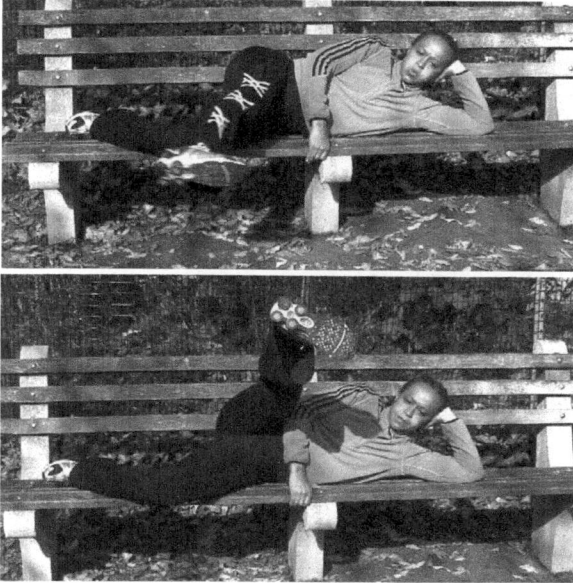

Action
- Lie on one side, legs slightly bent, supporting your head with your hand.
- Grab the front of the bench seat and slowly kick your upper leg out in front of you with a flexed foot.
- Lift the leg up as high as you can, moving your upper body as little as possible.
- Lower the leg down and kick back to starting position.
- Repeat as many times as you can.
- Switch sides.

Tips

- You'll be most comfortable on a bench with a flat seat and no back.
- Tone it down: Do just the forward and back kicks or the up and down kicks, rather than both.

35. Basic squat (moderate)

Squats are really a full body exercise that targets primarily your thigh, hip, and buttock muscles. But it will also engage the core muscles— back, abdomen, waist, and sides.

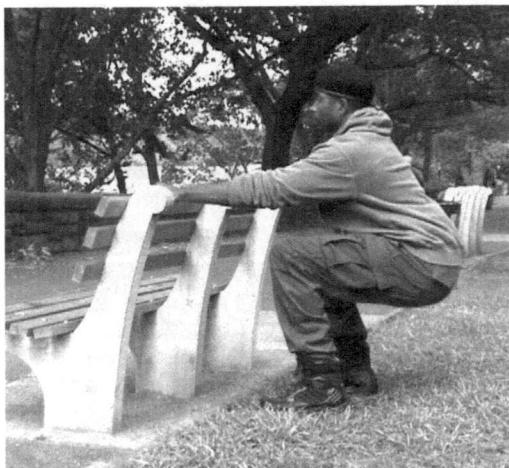

Action
- Stand tall, facing the back of the bench, with your feet parallel and hip-width apart.
- Place your hands lightly on the bench for support.
- Engage your core muscles, placing your weight back in your heels and bringing your hips back as you bend your knees, lowering your body into a squat until your thighs are parallel with the ground.
- Return to standing without locking your knees and repeat as many times as you can.

Tips

- Keep your shoulders relaxed and even, rather than allowing them to shrug up towards your ears.
- Keep your weight in your heels and your knees over your ankles.
- **+** Take it up a notch: Lower your body below parallel for a deeper squat, if this doesn't bother your knees.
- **−** Tone it down: Keep your knees less bent, so your thighs stay above parallel, for a shallower squat.

36. Squat and cross (moderate)

This combination movement gives you all the benefits of a squat plus a mini-abdominal workout thanks to the contraction needed to bring your knee in and over.

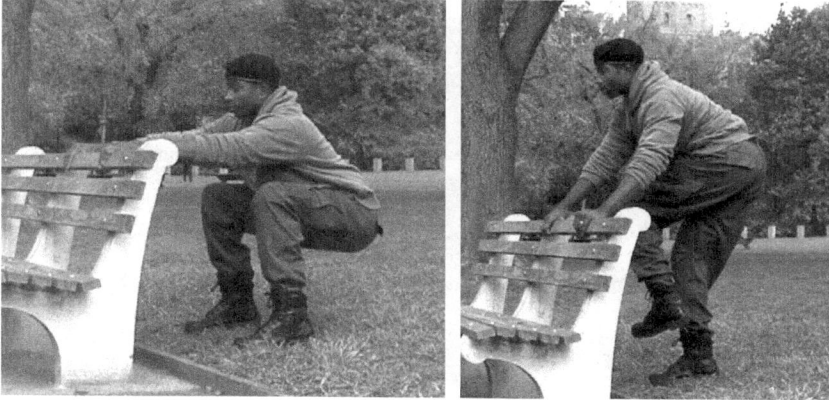

Action

- Stand tall, facing the back of the bench, feet parallel and hip-width apart.
- Place your hands lightly on the bench for support.
- Engage your core muscles, placing your weight back in your heels and bringing your hips back as you bend your knees, lowering your body into a squat until your thighs are parallel with the ground.
- As you rise up to a partial standing position, bring one knee towards the opposite shoulder.
- Place the foot back on the ground as you return to squatting position.
- Repeat, alternating legs, as many times as you can.

Tips

- Keep your shoulders relaxed and even, rather than allowing them to shrug up towards your ears.
- During the squat, keep your weight in your heels and your knees over your ankles.
- ✚ Take it up a notch: Lower your body below parallel for a deeper squat, if this doesn't bother your knees.
- ▬ Tone it down: Keep your knees less bent, so your thighs stay above parallel, for a shallower squat.

37. Tuck and kick (moderate)

The bigger the movement, the tighter and rounder your buttocks will be. So don't shortchange yourself—really tuck in that knee and extend that foot.

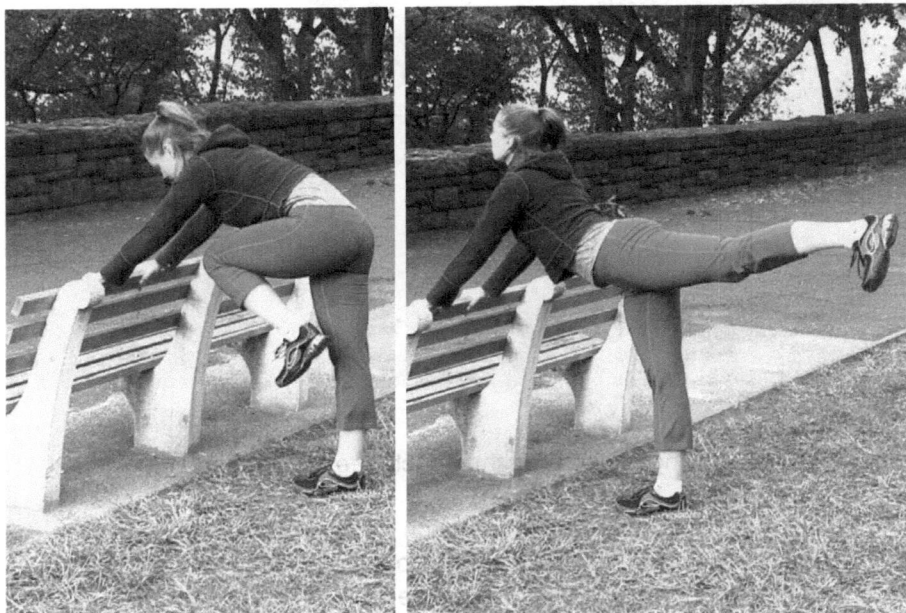

Action
- Stand tall behind the bench, feet together.
- Place both hands lightly on the bench back.
- Raise one leg behind you until it's at hip height.
- Bend your knee in towards your chest, and then extend it out.
- Repeat as many times as you can.
- Repeat with your other leg.

Tips

- Keep your body even, with both your hips on the same plane.
- Keep your shoulders relaxed and even, rather than allowing them to shrug up towards your ears.

➕ Take it up a notch: Let go of the bench, arms back, out to the side or in front of you for balance, while you tuck and extend your leg.

38. Sky kick (intense)

Okay, all you kickboxing fans. Check out this step-up with a high side kick. C'mon, give me some attitude and reach for the sky!

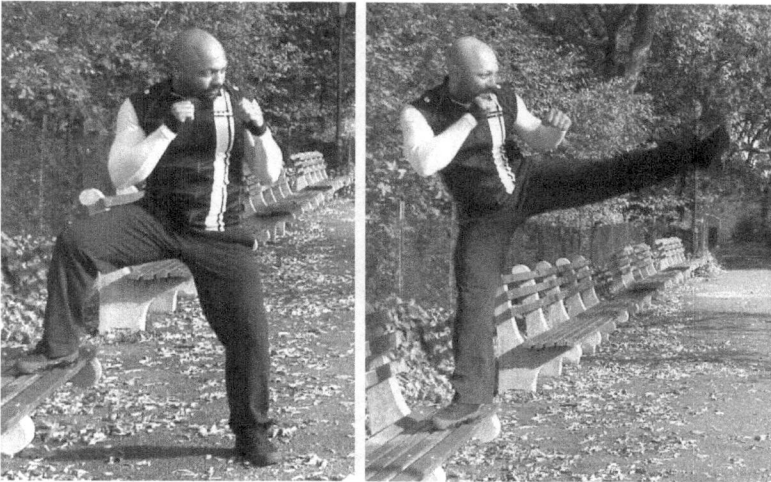

Action

- Stand with your side next to the bench, hands in loose fists near your chin.
- Side step up on the bench with your inner leg, as you bring your outer knee towards your chest, foot flexed.
- Immediately kick out to the side, about hip height, pushing forcefully with your heel.
- Retract the kick and return the outer leg to the ground and step down, bending the knee to protect your joints.
- Repeat with the same leg as many times as you can.
- Repeat on the other side.

Tips

- This is a martial arts move, so think of hitting a target with your kick.
- Try not to land with a crash when you step down—stay in control of the move.

+ Take it up a notch: Try adding a punch or two in between each kick.

– Tone it down: If doing this on the bench is too high for you, try this on the flat ground or on a small step or curb.

39. Xtreme knee lift (intense)

This may look familiar from step aerobics class, where it is known as "repeater." But the extra height of stepping up on a real bench makes it more extreme.

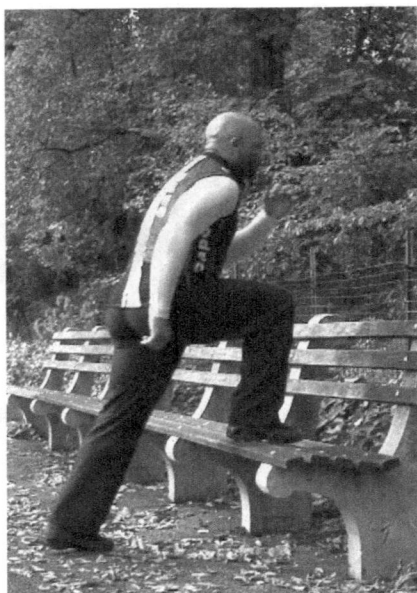

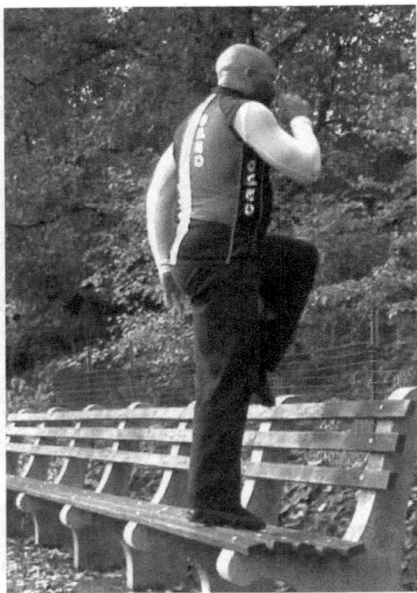

Action

- Face the bench and step up with the lead foot.
- Immediately bring the other knee up as high as you can in a knee lift.
- Step down with the same foot and immediately bring the knee up again.
- Repeat at least three times.
- Repeat with the other side.
- Continue alternating sides for the same number of repeats.

Tips

- Pump your arms in opposition to add momentum.
- Try not to land with a crash when you step down—stay in control of the move.
- — Tone it down: If a bench is too high for you, try this on the flat ground or on a small step or curb.

100

40. Split squat (intense)

Sometimes called a Bulgarian squat or a King squat, this is basically a one-legged lunge with your back foot on the bench to increase intensity. Hamstrings and buns watch out!

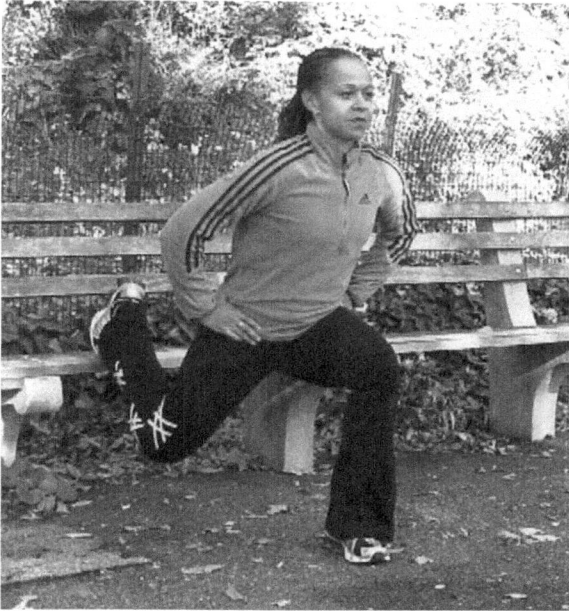

Action
• Stand tall a few feet away from the bench, facing away from the bench.
• Standing on one foot, lift the other foot onto the edge of the bench seat behind you, with the tops of your toes resting on the bench and your standing leg bent at a right angle, ankle.
• Place your hands on your hips.
• Bend and straighten your standing leg, driving your bodyweight into the heel of that foot.
• Repeat as many times as you can.
• Switch sides.

Tips

• Don't come all the way up; keep the knee slightly bent.
▬ Tone it down: If a bench is too high for you, try this on the flat ground or on a small step or curb.

101

41. Power jump (intense)

This exercise involves plyometrics, or explosive power moves, which help build strength, speed, and power. Swing your arms to give you momentum.

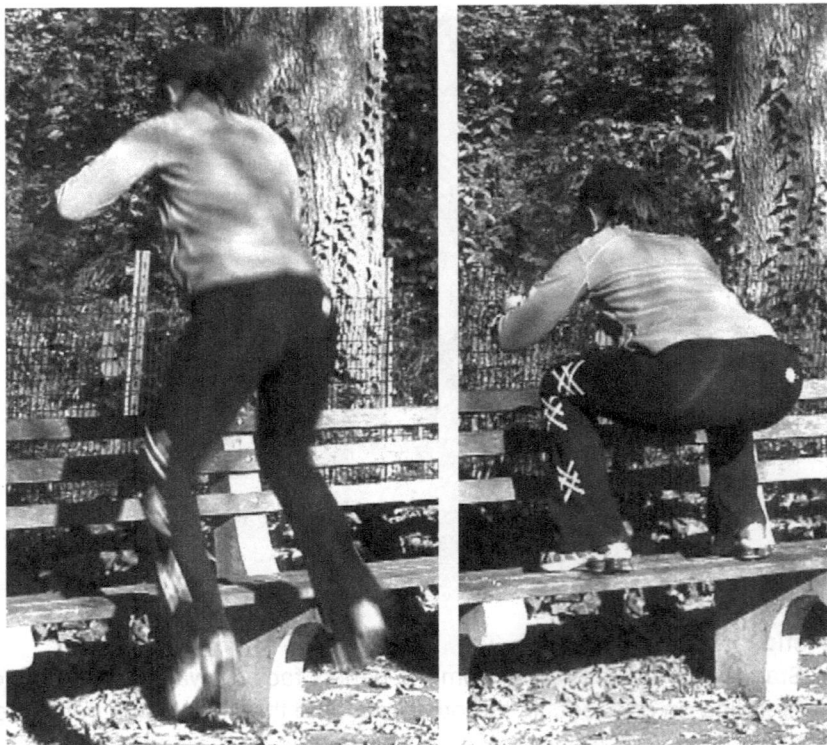

Action
- Face the bench, with feet at least hip-width apart.
- Squat down, bringing your arms back and forcefully jump up onto the bench seat, swinging your arms forward to help you.
- Step down and repeat as many times as you can.

Tips

- Use the momentum of swinging your arms to help you jump.
- If a bench is too high for you, try this on the flat ground or on a small step or curb.

102

42. Power taps (intense)

A great toner and strength builder for your legs and thighs, Power taps will also help your endurance if you work up to doing them long and fast enough.

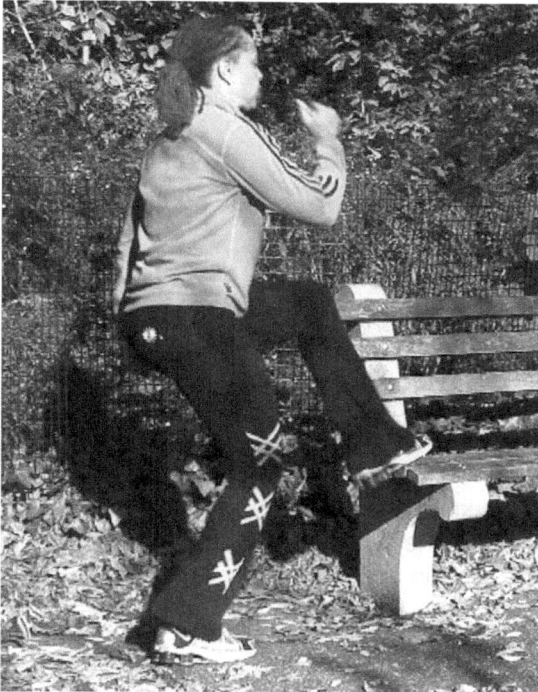

Action

- Standing tall, face the bench.
- Tap the edge of the bench seat with alternate feet, as if you were running in place.

Tips

- Use the momentum of your arms to keep you going.
- Start out by doing this slowly and building up speed as your fitness improves.
- **+** Take it up a notch: Increase your speed.
- **−** Tone it down: If a bench is too high for you, try this on a small step or curb.

43. One-legged squat (intense)

Just when you thought you knew all there was to know about squats! Try squatting while balancing on one leg at a time, with the height of the bench giving you extra depth and power.

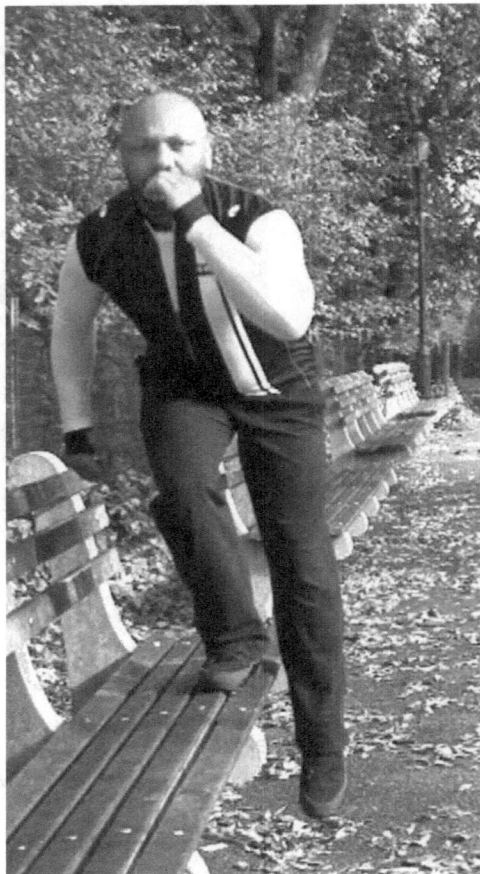

Action
- Stand with your side next to the bench.
- Side step up on the bench with your inner leg.
- Straighten up and stand on the leg that is on the bench, without locking the knee.
- Bend the standing knee, sinking the outer leg towards the ground without stepping on it, in a one-legged repetition.
- Do squats on the same leg as many times as you can.
- Repeat on the other side.

Tips

— Tone it down: Gently touch the ground with the outer leg during the squats. Or, if a bench is too high for you, try this on the flat ground or on a small step or curb.

104

CHAPTER THREE

Upper Body Strength

Women especially need to pay attention to their upper body's condition. We all want that flat stomach, but do you realize that a well-developed upper body is connected to your overall appearance, your posture—and the flatness of your tummy?

Did I mention resistance exercise can help with bat wings?

It is worth repeating the information provided in the section on lower body strength: well-developed muscles improve your metabolism, helping you lose fat, inches, and weight more easily, as well as maintain that sleek look. It's well accepted that "muscle dictates metabolism"—using resistance exercises to build your lean tissue, also known as muscle, burns more calories, even hours after you've finished exercising.

In this section, I give you over a dozen ways to sculpt and strengthen your shoulders, chest, and arms. And, no equipment other than your own body weight, gravity, and a park bench is required. Many of the exercises are in the push-up or plank family, and this means they are also working your core—and even your hips and legs. When you do them right, they work almost every muscle in your body. How great is that?

So, it's no wonder that push-ups are my absolutely favorite exercise. I often say to my followers: If you do ONE EXERCISE, this is the one. Women, don't groan. Men, don't moan. The push-up is infinitely adaptable to every level of fitness . . . it's not too simple or too boring or too difficult or too easy to perform. You won't need to cheat or ignore push-ups. We simply use the bench to modify the move. By switching up your hand and foot positions and adding in a few twists, the push-up becomes doable for some and a versatile muscle builder that will leave others begging for mercy. So, although you may equate push-ups with military-style workouts, or as a punishment in P.E. class, you're about to convert the push-up into your new best friend.

The rule is to train each major muscle group in your upper body two or three days each week using a variety of exercises. As mentioned previously, to make sure muscles have time to recover, wait at least 48 hours between resistance training exercises for a particular muscle group. The current recommendations are that you do 8-12 repetitions to improve strength and power, 10-15 repetitions to improve strength in middle-aged and older persons starting exercise, and 15-20 repetitions to improve muscular endurance. Or, if you're not the type who likes to keep track, there's a simpler way. Just repeat each exercise until you can't do any more ("muscle failure") and move on to the next exercise. You can do one "set" of repetitions, rest for a minute or so, and then do another set or two.

44. Modified push-up (light)

The usual way to make a push-up easier is to get down on your knees. Knee pain and knees stains are not necessary, when you have the bench to increase your leverage.

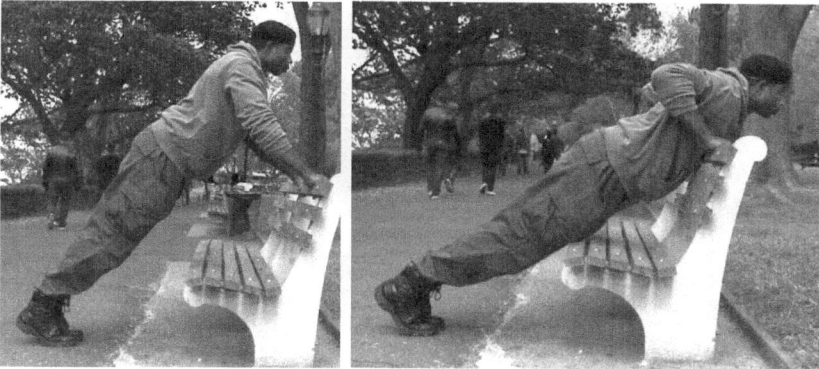

Action

- Place your hands on the bench back about shoulder-width apart, toes on the ground, heels raised.
- Tuck your hips under slightly and engage your abdominals, forming a straight line from the tip of your head to your feet. You may need to adjust the distance from your feet to the bench.
- Keeping your body straight, lower yourself all the way down so your chest lightly touches the bench. Your shoulders should be over your hands.
- Straighten your arms to push up away from the bench.
- Repeat as many times as you can, without losing your form.

Tips

- This is most comfortable on a bench with a rounded top edge.
- Vary the muscles you work by widening and narrowing your hand position. A wider grip targets the chest; a narrower one targets your triceps (the back of your arms).
- ➕ Take it up a notch: Place your hands on the bench seat instead of the back.
- ➖ Tone it down: Bend slightly at the hips ("pike position").

45. Pulsing push-up (moderate)

I sometimes call these "mini push-ups" because the action is so small. But the results are major!

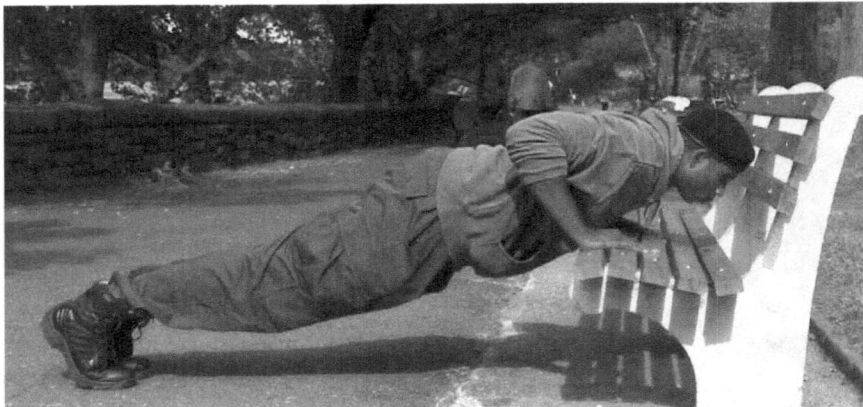

Action
- Place your hands on the bench seat about shoulder-width apart, toes on the ground, heels raised.
- Tuck your hips under slightly and engage your abdominals, forming a straight line from the tip of your head to your feet, shoulders over your hands. You may need to adjust the distance from your feet to the bench.
- Keeping your body straight, lower yourself all the way down so your chest lightly touches the bench.
- Straighten your arms slightly to push yourself one inch up, and then lower again.
- Continue to lower and raise your body for as many pulses as you can, without losing your form.

Tips

- Vary the muscles you work by widening and narrowing your hand position. A wider grip targets the chest; a narrower one targets your triceps.
- Tone it down: Bend slightly at the hips ("pike position") or place your hands on the back of the bench rather than the seat (one with a rounded top edge feels most comfortable.)

46. Push-off (moderate)

This push-up variation is a plyometric exercise—this style can help in-crease speed and explosiveness by loading and contracting a muscle as fast as possible. Plyometric exercises are particularly useful for ath-letes—but I like this one because a) I can actually do it, and b) it's so much fun to show off!

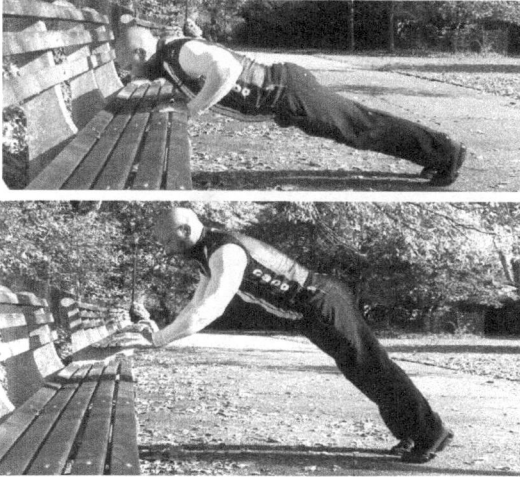

Action
- Place your hands on the bench seat about shoulder-width apart, toes on the ground, heels raised.
- Tuck your hips under slightly and engage your abdominals, forming a straight line from the tip of your head to your feet. You may need to adjust the distance from your feet to the bench.
- Keeping your body straight, lower yourself all the way down so your chest lightly touches the bench, shoulders over your hands.
- Push off the bench with enough force so your hands leave the bench for a moment before you catch yourself on the way down.
- Repeat for as many push-offs as you can, without losing your form.

Tips

— Tone it down: Place your hands on the back of the bench rather than the seat (one with a rounded top edge feels most comfortable).

47. Walking push-up (moderate)

Whenever my classes get a little stale in the push-up department, I switch to this variation. It totally wakes everyone up, and it can be done at any level of fitness.

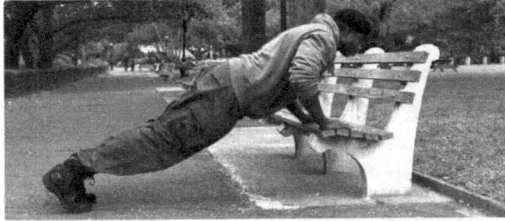

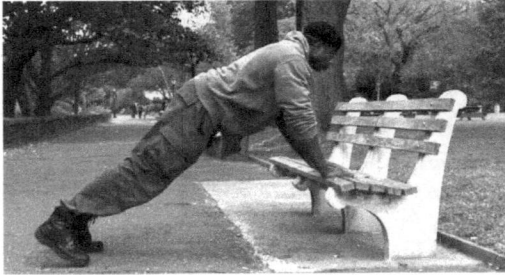

Action
- Start at one edge of the bench and place your hands on the bench seat about shoulder-width apart, toes on the ground, heels raised.
- Tuck your hips under slightly and engage your abdominals, forming a straight line from the tip of your head to your feet. You may need to adjust the distance from your feet to the bench.
- Keeping your body straight, lower yourself all the way down so your chest lightly touches the bench, shoulders over your hands.
- Push up to starting position and take a "step" with your hands and then your feet, moving towards the right or the left; repeat the push-up in your new position.
- Keep "walking" along the bench, alternating push-ups and "steps" until you reach the end of the bench. Then reverse direction.

Tips

− Tone it down: Bend slightly at the hips ("pike position") or place your hands on the back of the bench rather than on the seat (one with a rounded top edge feels most comfortable).

110

48. Push-off and clap (moderate)

The clapping push-up is the same thing as a plyometric push-up or push-off (#46). The only difference is that when you explode off the bench, you clap your hands while you're in the air. And it looks even cooler.

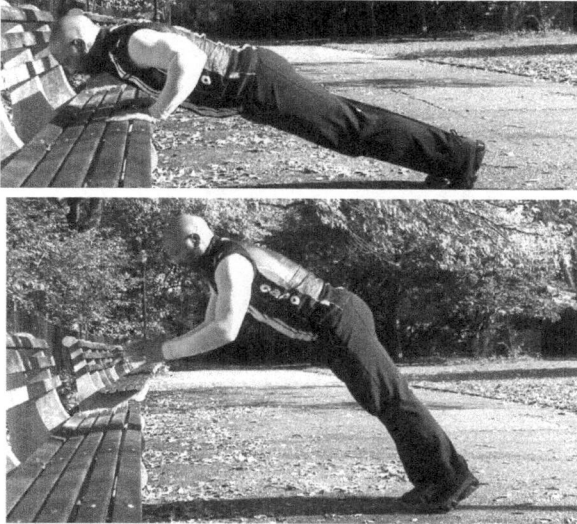

Action

- Place your hands on the bench back or seat about shoulder-width apart. Tuck your hips under and engage your abdominals.
- Keeping your body straight, lower yourself all the way down so your chest lightly touches the bench.
- Push off the bench with enough force so your hands leave the bench; clap your hands together in the air before you catch yourself on the way down.
- Repeat for as many push-offs as you can, without losing your form and still being able to clap between each repetition.

Tips

+ Take it up a notch: Try the triple clap push-up: As your body is coming up, clap once, when your body reaches its peak, clap behind your back, and before your hands hit the bench, clap one more time. Yee-hah!

– Tone it down: Place your hands on the back of the bench rather than the seat (one with a rounded top edge feels most comfortable).

49. Side plank and arm circle (moderate)

This side plank variation combines strength and flexibility. It's a beautiful thing.

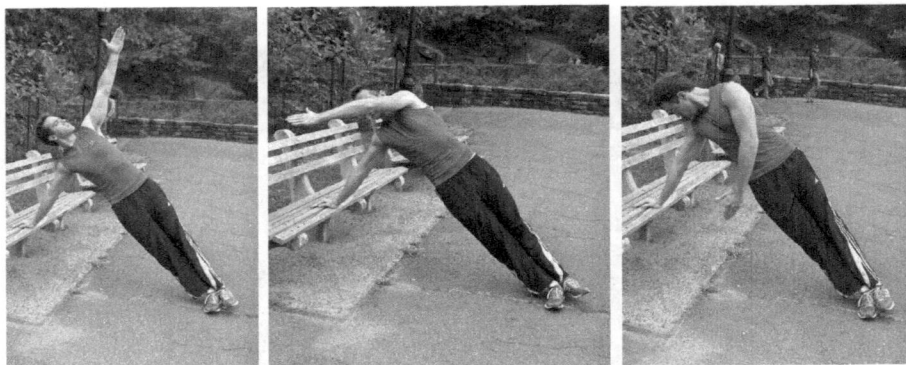

Action
- Stand with your side to the bench, feet crossed over one another, parallel on the ground and a good distance away from the bench, so your body is in a straight line when you're leaning on the bench.
- Place your inside hand on the bench seat, hips stacked on top of one another.
- Sweep your outer hand out, up, around and down in a circle.
- Repeat as many times as you can; reverse direction.
- Switch sides and repeat with your other arm.

Tips

- Hold your torso steady, contracting your abdominals, making sure your hips don't sink down.
- As it makes the circle, follow your hand with your gaze.
- ✚ Take it up a notch: Stack one foot on top of the other, or lift your outer foot off the ground.
- ▬ Tone it down: Place your hands on the back of the bench rather than the seat (one with a rounded top edge feels most comfortable).

50. Walk the plank (light)

I've borrowed this idea from yoga, where we sometimes jump back from a forward bend to a plank and then back up again. The Nancercize variation allows you to walk the distance instead of jumping; having your hands on the bench instead of the ground also makes it more do-able for more people.

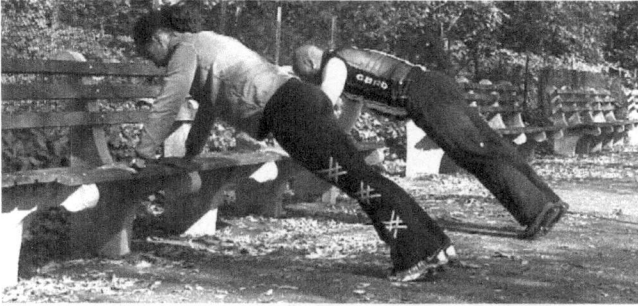

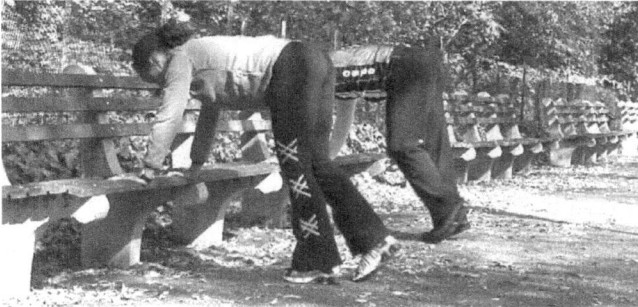

Action
- Stand tall, facing the bench. Place your hands on the bench seat, shoulder-width apart; be on your toes with heels raised.
- Taking 3-4 steps, walk your feet towards the bench, and then away from the bench.
- Repeat as many times as you can.

Tips

➕ Take it up a notch: For a more intense arm workout as well as an aerobic aspect, replace some or all of the walking steps with a jump.
➖ Tone it down: Place your hands on the back of the bench rather than the seat (one with a rounded top edge feels most comfortable).

113

51. Leg lift push-up (moderate)

The leg lift push-up works your core and gluteus in addition to your upper body. Having one leg up in the air and off the ground puts more weight on your upper body, forcing it to work harder.

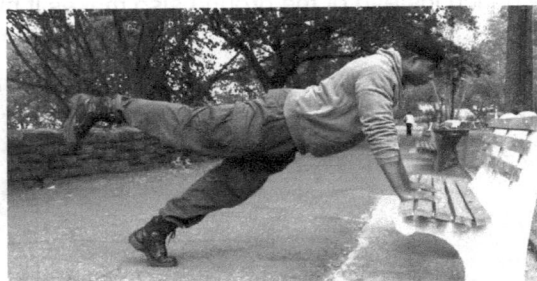

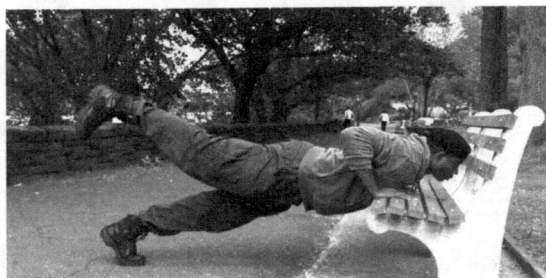

Action
- Place your hands on the bench seat about shoulder-width apart, toes on the ground, heels raised.
- Tuck your hips under slightly and engage your abdominals, forming a straight line from the tip of your head to your feet. You may need to adjust the distance from your feet to the bench.
- Lift one leg so it is level with your hips, and balance your weight on the other foot.
- Keeping your body straight, lower yourself all the way down so your chest lightly touches the bench, shoulders over your hands.
- Do as many push-ups as you can, then repeat with the other leg raised.

Tips

— Tone it down: Place your hands on the back of the bench rather than the seat (one with a rounded top edge feels most comfortable).

52. Basic dip (light)

Nothing beats dips for working the back of your arms, chest, and shoulders. The other wonderful thing is, these moves are so subtle you can easily sneak 10 basic dips without anyone noticing!

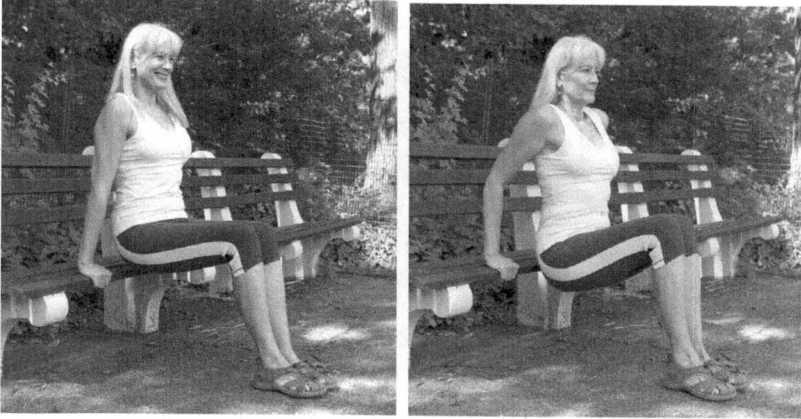

Action

- Sit on the bench, hands on either side of you, thumbs touching your hips.
- Place your feet together or hip-width apart on the ground in front of you.
- Press down on your hands and lift your torso off the bench, elongating it and bringing your hips forward, just in front of the bench seat. You may need to adjust your feet a bit.
- Bend your elbows and lower your hips, keeping them close to the bench.
- Push back up, straightening your arms, doing as many repetitions as you can.

Tips

- Keep your shoulders down and away from your ears.
- Avoid locking your elbows when you push up, or bending beyond 90 degrees.

➕ Take it up a notch: Do the dips with your feet farther away from the bench or even with straight legs.

➖ Tone it down: Once you lift your torso off the bench, just hold it there for as long as you can, without bending your elbows, for an isometric contraction.

53. Cross-legged dip (moderate)

When you need a change from basic dips, the cross-legged dip comes to the rescue. This is also a bit more difficult than the basic dip because more of your weight is supported by your upper body. It also gives your hips a nice stretch!

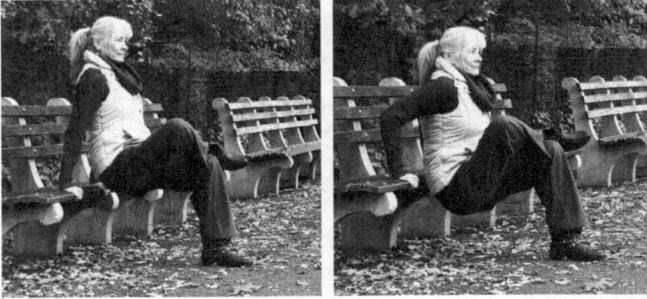

Action
- Sit on the bench, hands on either side of you, thumbs touching your hips.
- Place your feet hip-width apart on the ground in front of you.
- Cross the ankle of one leg over the knee of the other.
- Press down on your hands and lift your torso off the bench, elongating it and bringing your hips forward, just in front of the bench seat. You may need to adjust your feet a bit.
- Bend your elbows and lower your hips, keeping them close to the bench.
- Push back up, straightening your arms, doing as many repetitions as you can.
- Switch legs and repeat.

Tips

- Keep your shoulders down and away from your ears.
- Avoid locking your elbows when you push up, or bending beyond 90 degrees.

+ Take it up a notch: Do the dips with your feet farther away from the bench or even with straight legs.

– Tone it down: Once you lift your torso off the bench, just hold it there for as long as you can, without bending your elbows, for an isometric contraction.

116

54. One-legged dip (moderate)

This also adds zip to the basic dip. It's more strenuous due to the shift in weight from two legs to one, and you're also working your core more by keeping one leg extended in front of you.

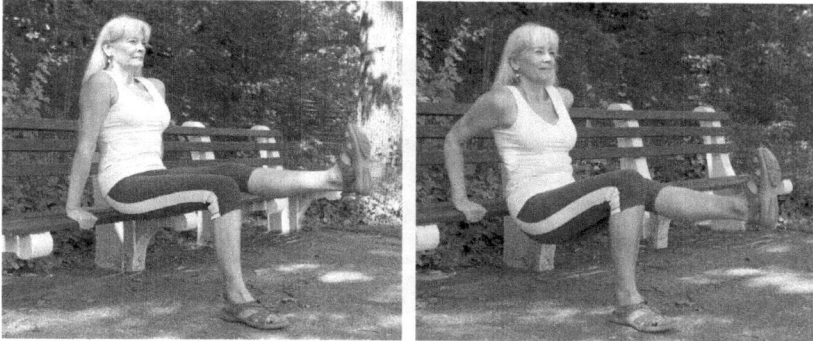

Action

- Sit on the bench, hands on either side of you, thumbs touching your hips.
- Place your feet hip-width apart on the ground in front of you.
- Lift one leg off the ground until it is even with your other thigh.
- Press down on your hands and lift your torso off the bench, elongating it and bringing your hips forward, just in front of the bench seat. You may need to adjust your feet a bit.
- Bend your elbows and lower your hips, keeping them close to the bench.
- Push back up, straightening your arms, doing as many repetitions as you can.
- Switch legs and repeat.

Tips

- Keep your shoulders down and away from your ears.
- Avoid locking your elbows when you push up, or bending beyond 90 degrees.

➕ Take it up a notch: Do the dips with your feet farther away from the bench or even with straight legs.

➖ Tone it down: Once you lift your torso off the bench, just hold it there for as long as you can, without bending your elbows, for an isometric contraction.

55. One-arm triceps push-up (intense)

Amateurs need not apply! You'll be lifting your body weight using just the little ole triceps muscle of one arm. A real challenge, but bye-bye batwings.

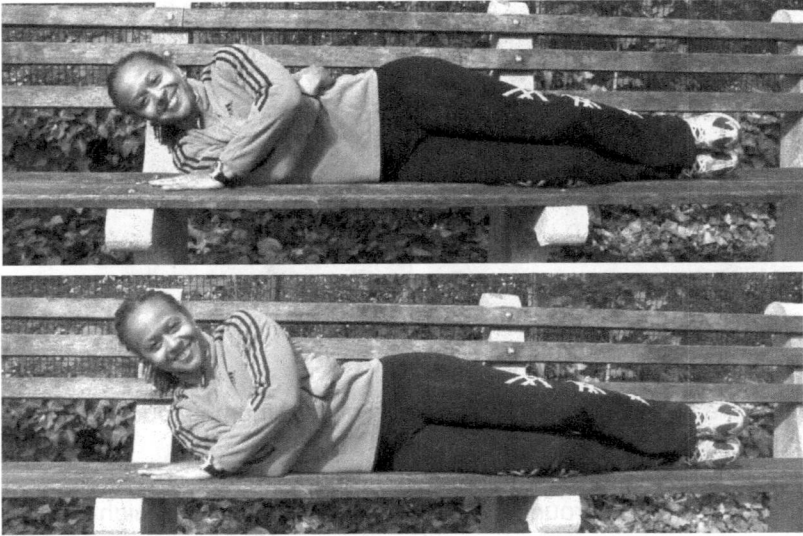

Action

- Lie on the bench on your side with both knees bent and your hips stacked on top of one another.
- Wrap your inside arm around your waist and place your outside hand on the bench in front of you, palm flat.
- Press down with your outside hand to push your upper body up and off the bench, straightening your working arm as much as you can without locking the elbow.
- Lower your body down a few inches and repeat pushing up and down for as many times as you can.
- Switch sides and repeat with your other arm.

Tips

- This will feel best on a bench that has a flat seat, and you might prefer the extra freedom of a backless bench.

118

56. Power push-up (intense)

If a standard push-up has gotten a little ho-hum, or if you just want to take it to the next level and impress the squirrels, try elevating your feet on the bench. Oh, and it will work those beautiful shoulders a bit more, too.

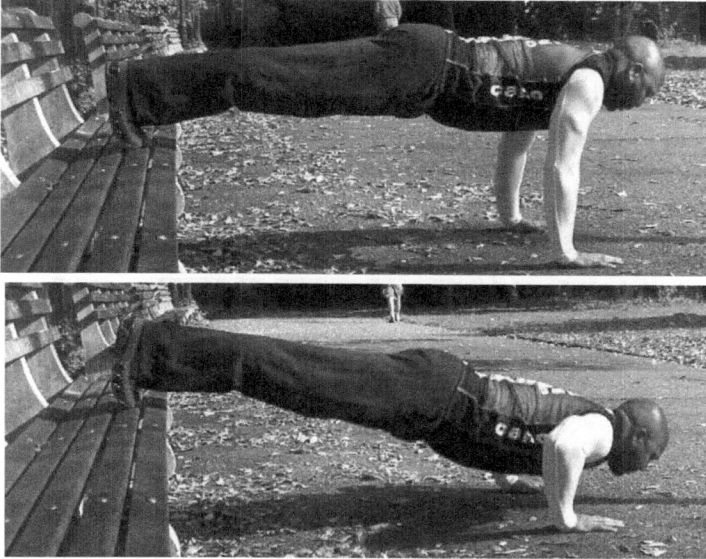

Action
- Place your hands on the ground and your feet on the edge of the bench seat about shoulder-width apart. Tuck your hips under and engage your abdominals.
- Keeping your body straight from head to toe, lower yourself down so your chest almost touches the ground.
- Straighten your arms to push yourself up, and then lower yourself again.
- Continue to lower and raise your body for as many times as you can, without losing your form.

Tips

- Mix up the muscles you work by widening and narrowing your hand position. A wider grip targets the chest; a narrower one targets your triceps.
- ➕ Take it up a notch: Place your feet on the bench back or just hold it in the down position for as long as you can.

119

57. One-arm power push-up (intense)

No doubt about it, this one's a killer. You need a lot of strength in your arms, shoulders, and chest as well the ability to engage several smaller muscles to stabilize yourself as you lift and lower your bodyweight using just one arm. It's a move that will definitely impress any passers-by!

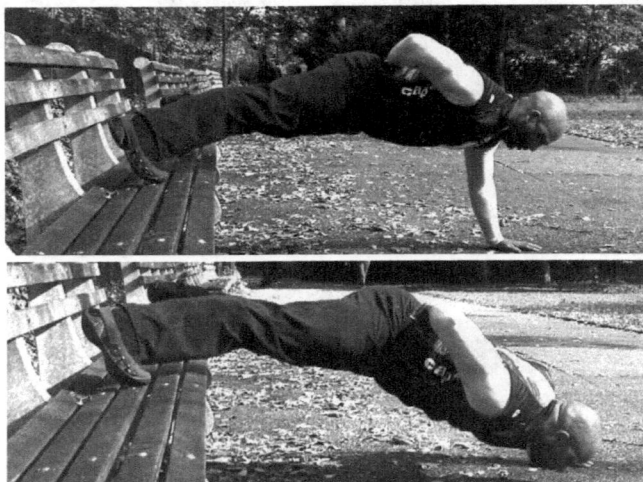

Action

- Place your hands on the ground and your feet on bench seat wider than shoulder-width apart. Tuck your hips under and engage your abdominals.
- Place one hand behind your back.
- Keeping your body straight, lower yourself down so your head almost touches the ground.
- Straighten your arm to push yourself up, and then lower again.
- Continue to lower and raise your body for as many times as you can, without losing your form.
- Then switch to the other arm.

Tips

- Work your way up by starting on the ground and then a short curb before progressing to the bench.
- Tone it down: Turn your torso and legs slightly away from the pressing hand.

120

58. Handstand push-up (intense)

Okay, this is actually the modified version—in the standard version, you're actually doing a full handstand. Still, it helps if you're playing the theme from *Rocky* in your head when you do these.

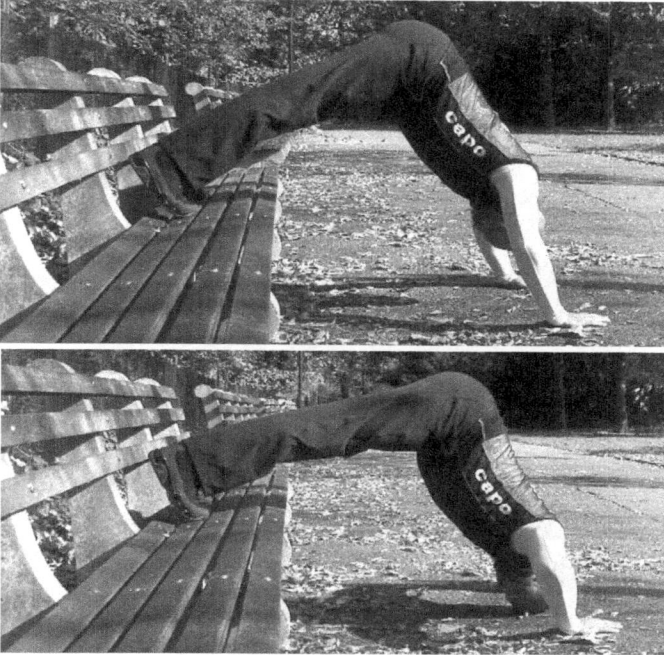

Action
- Place your hands on the ground and your feet on the bench seat shoulder-width apart, forming an inverted V shape.
- Lower yourself down until your head almost touches the ground.
- Straighten your arms to push yourself up, and then lower again.
- Continue to lower and raise your body for as many times as you can, without losing your form.

Tips

➕ Take it up a notch: Place your feet on the bench back instead of the seat.

59. Wheelbarrow (intense)

When I was a kid, this was a favorite game. We took turns holding each other's feet and walking across the grass. Little did we know what a great workout we were getting.

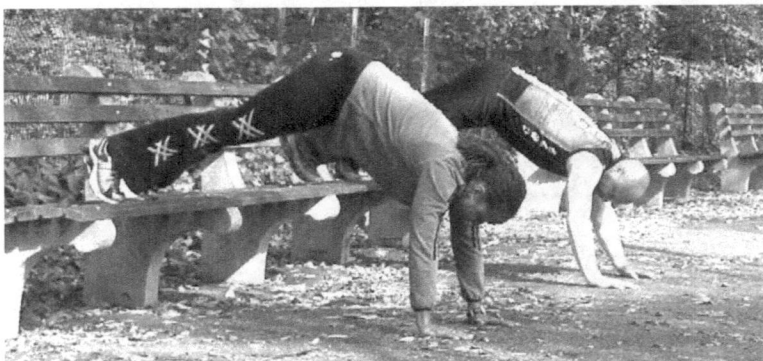

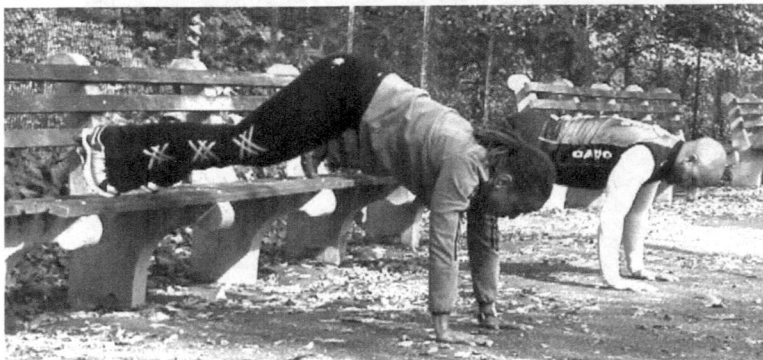

Action
- Place your hands on the ground and your feet on the bench seat, shoulder-width apart, forming an inverted V shape.
- Walk your hands out until you are parallel to the ground.
- Walk your hands back to the starting position.

Tips

➕ Take it up a notch: Place your feet on the back of the bench.
➖ Tone it down: Stop short of walking your hands all the way out.

122

CHAPTER FOUR

Core Strength

What is your core and why should you care about it? "Core" is the word that fitness trainers use to cover all the muscles in your middle. So, an in-shape core is needed for a firm, flat belly—something we all pretty much want. But there's so much more to our core than that, and so many other exercises to do besides endless sit-ups and crunches!

Your core is actually where all movement in your body originates—it includes the muscles in your pelvis, lower back, hips, and abdomen. When these are strong and work harmoniously together, you not only look better, you also have better balance and stability. Are you beginning to see how your core really is central to just about everything you do in life—from picking a flower to reaching a vase on the top shelf, from shoveling snow to dancing a tango?

On the other hand, a weak core can lead to poor posture, lower back pain, and muscle injuries. Strong core muscles provide the brace of support needed to help prevent such pain and injury.

To work your core most effectively, you need to come at it from many angles, and in this section, I show you a wide variety of ways to do just that. For example, you'll find surprising twists on familiar exercises like the sit-up and the bicycle. As is the case with upper body strengthening in the previous section, a lot of core work depends on doing a plank correctly. And, since your core needs to be working to do just about ANY movement, if you find you're having problems performing the exercises in the other sections of this book, it might be because your core is weak.

Remember, although a strong core will help, core exercises alone won't give you a flat belly if you have a layer of fat on top of your tummy muscles, no matter how toned. You also need to watch what you eat and perform full body workouts, where you exercise all your muscle groups, burn calories and fat, and boost your metabolism.

Core Strength

Generally, you can work your core muscles everyday; if you do, it makes sense to vary your choices!

60. Basic sit-up (moderate)

This version of the sit-up is actually easier than the standard floor sit-up because the bench back helps keep your thighs from flying up. This one is most fun with a buddy so you can alternate who's going up and who's going down. Or you can do this in sync and compete to see who can do the most.

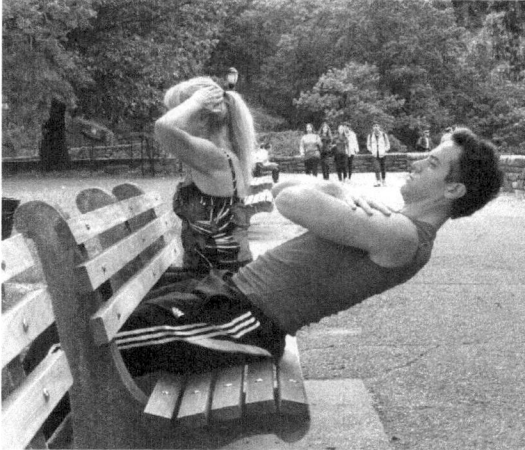

Action

- Sit tall on the bench facing the back and slide both legs in the space between the bench seat and back.
- Place your hands at the back or side of your head, elbows out, or crossed over your chest.
- Exhale and contract your abdominal muscles as you slowly lower your torso down behind you as far as you can comfortably go.
- Contract your abs to lift your torso and curl up. Imagine you are squeezing your belly button to your spine.
- Do as many repetitions as you can.

Tips

- You may be more comfortable on a bench with a flat rather than a curved seat and, If the space is narrow for your thighs, on a bench with no back.
- ➕ Take it up a notch: Pause when your torso reaches the lowest point.
- ➖ Tone it down: Lower your torso less.

61. Hug yourself and twist (moderate)

This exercise works the front abdominal muscles as well as the sides of your waist. Rotation exercises like this reach deep into the core muscles surrounding and supporting your spine.

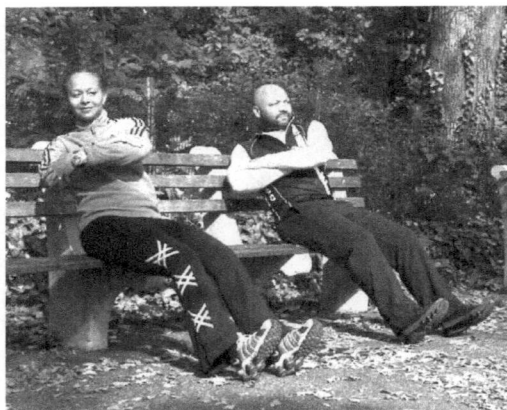

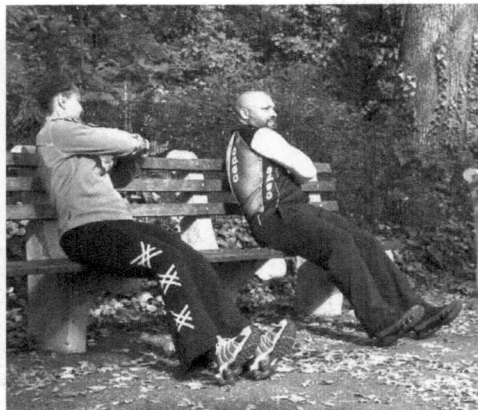

Action
- Sit on the edge of the bench, heels on the ground, with your arms crossed over your chest, each hand holding the opposite elbow.
- Contract your abdominal muscles and lean so your back is almost touching the back of the bench.
- Staying angled back, twist slowly from side to side, rotating your entire torso, not just your arms.
- Do as many twists as you can.

Tips

- You may be more comfortable on a bench that has a flat seat, rather than a curved one.

➕ Take it up a notch: Do this on a bench with no back and lean back farther.

➖ Tone it down: Lightly rest your back on the bench for support until you get stronger.

126

62. Hippy dippy plank (moderate)

Despite the silly name I've given it, this exercise is serious business. The hip dip and lift is a true challenge for your oblique abdominal muscles (on the side), which can sometimes be a difficult part of the core to reach.

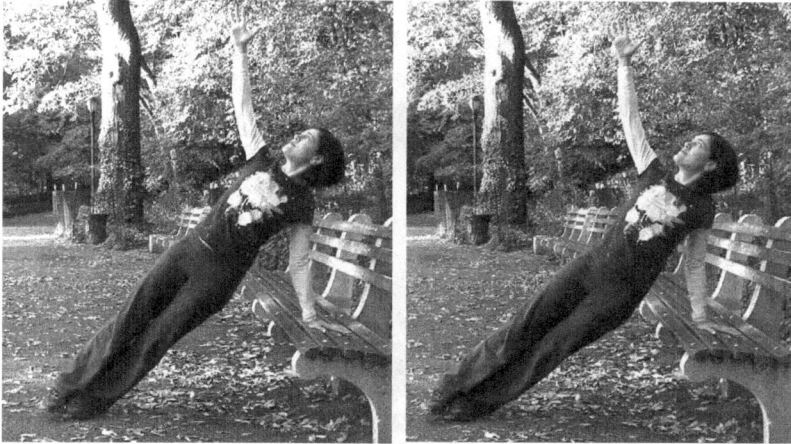

Action

- Standing tall with your side to the bench, place your inside hand on the bench seat, palm down, directly under your shoulder.
- Stack your feet on top of one another or cross one in front of the other.
- Contract your core and buttocks and raise your hips so they form a straight line from your feet to your shoulders as you reach up with the outside arm and look up at it.
- Lower your inside hip towards the ground a few inches.
- Lift your hips back up and repeat as many times as you can, maintaining the straight line of your body.
- Switch sides and repeat.

Tips

- Avoid sinking into your shoulder and keep your neck long.
- You may find it easier to balance if you look straight ahead rather than at your raised hand.
- ✚ Take it up a notch: Balance on your forearm instead of your hand.
- ➖ Tone it down: Place your hand on the bench back instead of the seat.

63. Basic bicycle (moderate)

This oldie but goodie hits all of your abdominal muscles, but in particular the lower abdominals. You will feel the burn, but in a good way.

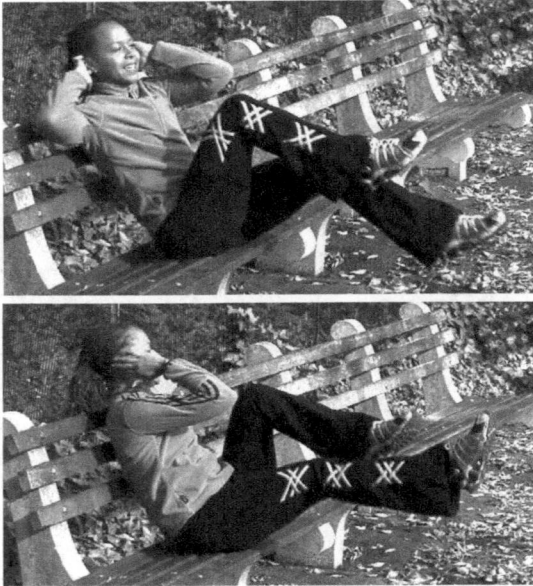

Action
- Sit on the bench, near the edge, and place your hands at the back or side of your head.
- Lean so your back is almost touching the back of the bench.
- Bring one knee up towards the opposite elbow, trying to touch it.
- Switch and bring your other leg to the opposite elbow.
- Do as many repetitions as you can, smoothly and rhythmically alternating legs, as if you were on a bicycle.

Tips

- You may be more comfortable on a bench that has a flat seat, rather than a curved one.
- **+** Take it up a notch: Do this very slowly. Or do it really fast.
- **−** Tone it down: Let your foot lightly touch the ground as the other one comes up, or rest your back on the bench.

64. Modified plank (light)

The plank is a great way to build up your strength and endurance in almost every muscle of your body, but the accent is on the core muscles of your abs and back. I've included a lot of variations in this chapter, but the modified plank is a great place to start.

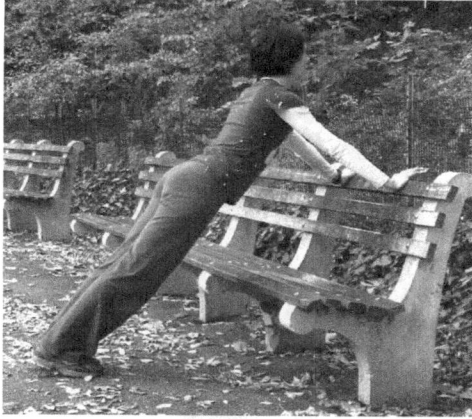

Action

- Standing tall, face the bench and place your hands on the bench back, standing with your heels on the ground, or on your toes, whichever is most comfortable.
- Keep your back flat, with your hips a bit tucked and abdomen contracted, forming a straight line from your feet to your head.
- Hold this position, inhaling and exhaling, for as long as you can (for up to one minute and at least 10-30 seconds).

Tips

- This may feel most comfortable on a bench back with a rounded top edge.
- Keep shoulders down and away from your ears, and your head in line with your spine, eyes gazing ahead of you.
- Don't let your hips sink down—think of your body as, well, a plank.
- ➕ To increase the intensity slightly, try this with your hands on the bench seat, palms directly under your shoulders. Or, raise your left arm so it points to 10 o'clock and hold; lower it and raise your right hand to 2 o'clock and hold; keep alternating for as long as you can.

129

65. Double leg lift (intense)

You may recognize this from Pilates. It's extremely simple, but challenging to do correctly.

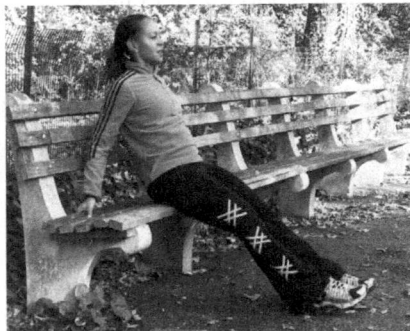

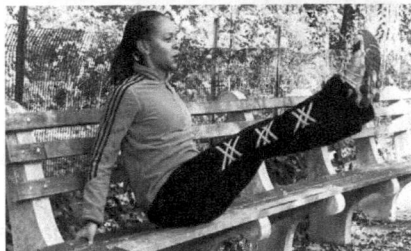

Action

- Sit on the edge of the bench, legs straight out in front of you, feet resting on the ground. Lean so your back is almost touching the back of the bench.
- Grab the rear edge of the seat for support; contract your abdominal muscles and lift both legs up as high as you can.
- Slowly lower both legs down, tapping the ground slightly, and immediately lift your legs back up again.
- Repeat as many times as you can.

Tips

- A bench with a flat seat is the most comfortable one for this position. It may be tempting to hold your breath, but be sure to inhale and exhale rhythmically.

➕ Take it up a notch: Let go of the bench and place your hands behind your head.

➖ Tone it down: Lift only one leg at a time.

130

66. Scissor kick (intense)

This is a relatively small movement, but when you do Scissor kicks, you tremendously isolate your lower abdominal muscles.

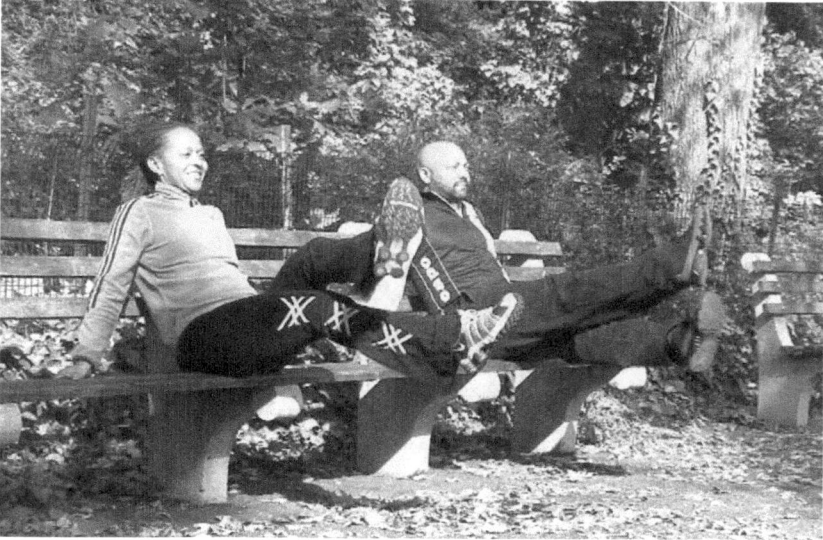

Action
- Sit on the edge of the bench, legs straight out in front of you, feet resting on the ground.
- Lean so your back is almost touching the back of the bench.
- Grab the rear edge of the seat for support; contract your abdominal muscles and lift both legs up as high as you can.
- Separate your feet about one foot apart and then cross one over the other, in a scissors motion.
- Repeat, alternating feet, as many times as you can.

Tips

- It may be tempting to hold your breath, but be sure to inhale and exhale rhythmically.
- A bench with a flat seat is the most comfortable one for this position.
- ➕ Take it up a notch: Let go of the bench and place your hands behind your head.
- ➖ Tone it down: Bend your knees slightly.

131

67. Flutter kick (intense)

The Flutter is similar to the Scissor kick but strengthens the hip flexor muscles like crazy. Be sure to stretch your thighs and hips after this one.

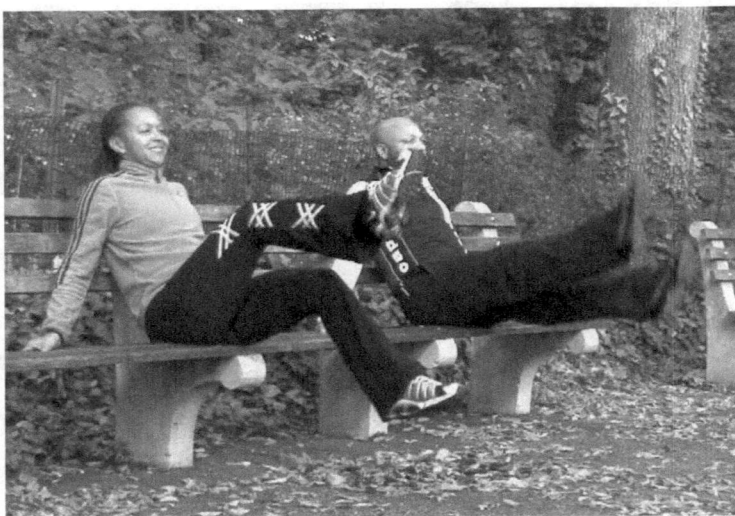

Action
- Sit on the edge of the bench, legs straight out in front of you, feet resting on the ground.
- Lean so your back is almost touching the back of the bench.
- Grab the rear edge of the seat for support; contract your abdominal muscles and lift both legs up as high as you can.
- Drop one foot a few inches toward the ground and lift it up again, then drop the other foot and lift up again in a flutter motion.
- Repeat as many times as you can.

Tips

- A bench with a flat seat is the most comfortable one for this position.
- It may be tempting to hold your breath, but be sure to inhale and exhale rhythmically.

+ Take it up a notch: Let go of the bench and place your hands behind your head.

– Tone it down: Bend your knees slightly, and tap your foot lightly on the ground on the downswing.

132

68. Roll up (moderate)

Keeping your knees bent while raising your hips targets your lower and middle abdominal muscles, as well as your upper thighs and lower back. The behind-the-head bench grab improves flexibility and strength in your upper body too.

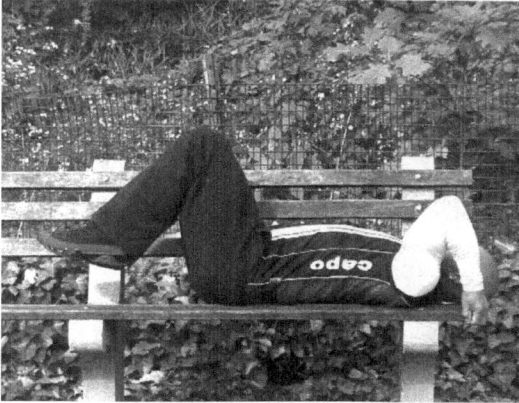

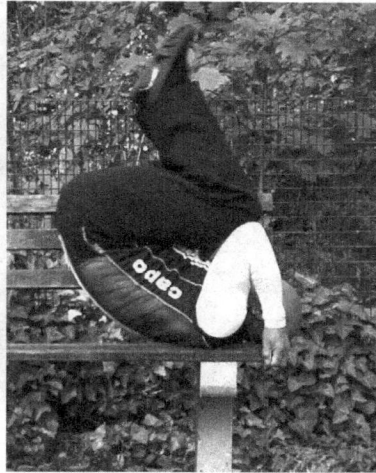

Action
- Lie on the bench with your head near one end, and with your knees bent.
- Reach over your head and grab the edge of the bench for support.
- Contract your abdominal muscles and bring your knees towards your chest.
- Contract even more and curl your hips off the bench, rolling onto your shoulders and reaching your knees towards your head.
- Curl back down and repeat as many times as you can.

Tips

- A bench with a flat seat will be most comfortable.
- — Tone it down: do a more moderate roll, stopping before you roll all the way onto your shoulders.

133

69. Hip lift (moderate)

You'll feel this really hit the muscles between your ribs and your hips, as well as those running along the side of your torso

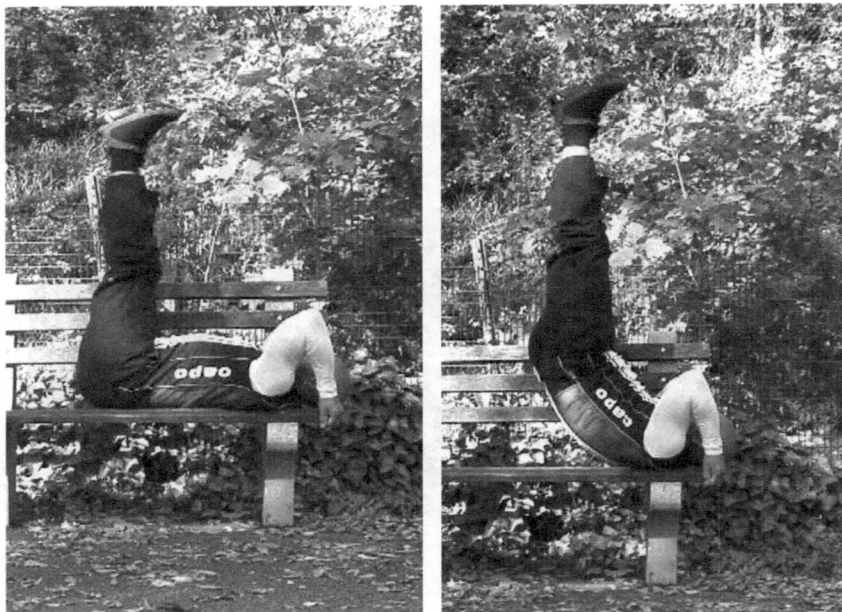

Action

- Lie on the bench with your head near one end, and your legs straight up over your hips, perpendicular to the ground.
- Reach over your head and grab the edge of the bench for support.
- Contract your abdominal muscles and lift your hips and lower back off the bench, reaching your toes towards the sky.
- Lower back down slowly and smoothly and repeat as many times as you can.

Tips

- A bench with a flat seat will be most comfortable.
- — Tone it down: Only lift up a few inches before you come back down.

134

70. Elbow plank (moderate)

This may look like you're doing nothing . . . but come talk to me after you've held this for a full minute so I can hear how your abdominal muscles are complaining.

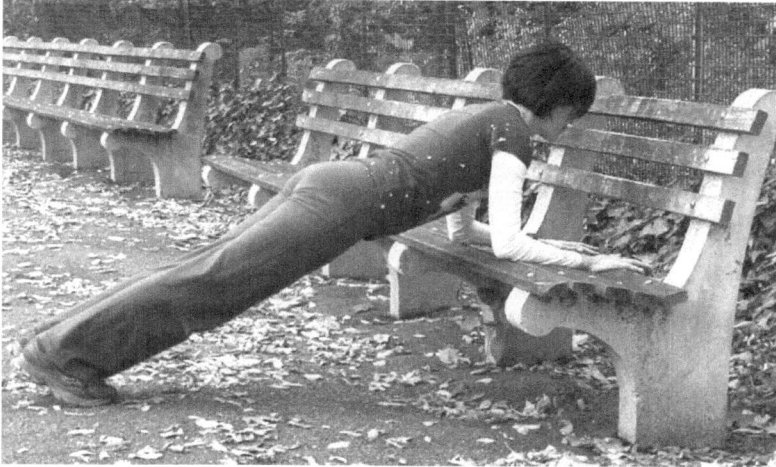

Action
- Standing tall, face the bench and place your forearms on the bench seat, your elbows directly under your shoulders.
- Extend your legs back, toes on the ground and close together.
- Keep your back flat, with your hips a bit tucked and abdomen contracted, creating a straight line with your body from feet to head.
- Hold this position, inhaling and exhaling, for as long as you can (at last 10-30 seconds and up to one minute).

Tips

- This may feel most comfortable on a bench seat that is flat rather than rounded.
- Keep your shoulders down and away from your ears, and your head in line with your spine, eyes gazing ahead of you.
- Avoid sinking into your shoulders or letting your hips or head drop down.
- — Tone it down: bend slightly at the hips, forming an inverted V shape with your legs and torso ("pike" position).

135

71. Knee drop plank (moderate)

Another unflamboyant variation of the yoga plank position. All the work is going on deep inside, to strengthen your front, back, and side muscles.

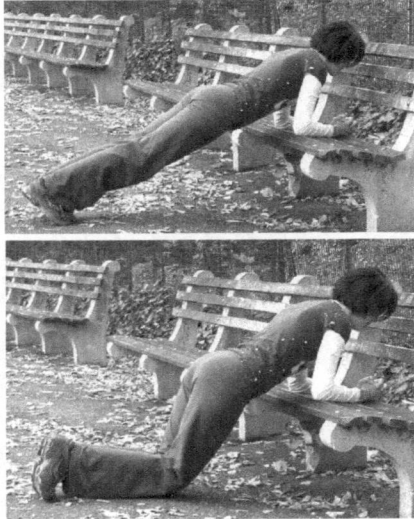

Action

- Standing tall, face the bench and place your forearms on the bench seat, your elbows directly under your shoulders.
- Extend your legs back, toes on the ground and close together.
- Keep your back flat, with your hips a bit tucked and abdomen contracted, your body a straight line from heel to head.
- Bend your knees towards the ground, keeping the rest of your body firm and in place; let your knees hover a few inches off the ground for a moment.
- Straighten your legs back to starting position and hold for a moment; repeat slowly as many times as you can.

Tips

- This may feel most comfortable on a bench seat that is flat rather than rounded.
- Keep your shoulders down and away from your ears, and your head in line with your spine, eyes gazing ahead of you.

72. Air pump (light)

This variation on a classic Pilates floor exercise called the Hundred works just as well on a bench outdoors. It's often used as a warm-up at the beginning of a series of core exercises.

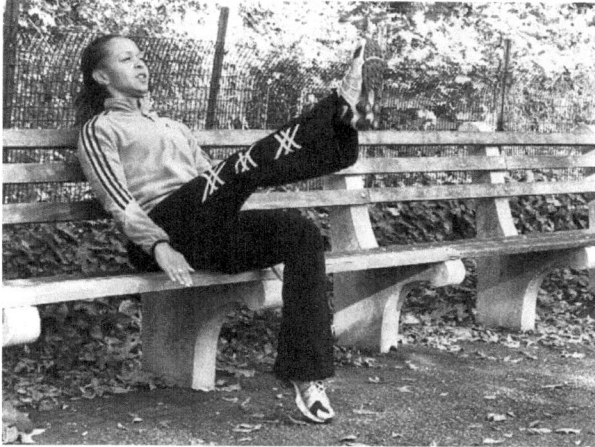

Action

- Sit on the bench with both feet on the ground; lean so your back is almost touching the back of the bench, and your abdominal muscles stay engaged to the utmost.
- Lift one leg up as high as you can, keeping it as straight as you can, while your other foot stays lightly on the ground.
- Pump your arms up and down for a few inhales and exhales as you hold your raised leg steady.
- Switch legs and pump your arms for a few inhales and exhales.
- Repeat, alternating legs, for as long as you can—the goal is 100 pumps.

Tips

- A bench with a flat seat is the most comfortable one for this position.
- It may be tempting to hold your breath, but be sure to inhale and exhale rhythmically in coordination with the arm pumps.
- **+** Take it up a notch: Raise both legs as you pump.
- **−** Tone it down: Place both feet on the ground as you pump, or rest your back on the bench back.

73. Coasting bicycle (moderate)

Unlike coasting on a bicycle, you won't be resting during the "hold" position. The bicycle is a type of crunch that works the entire abdominal family.

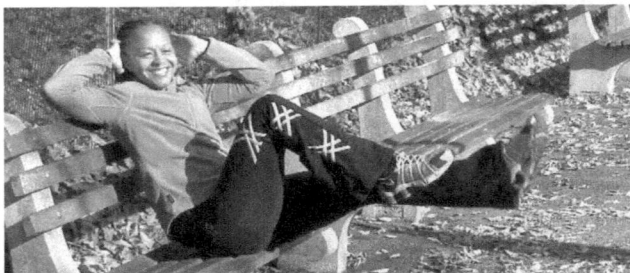

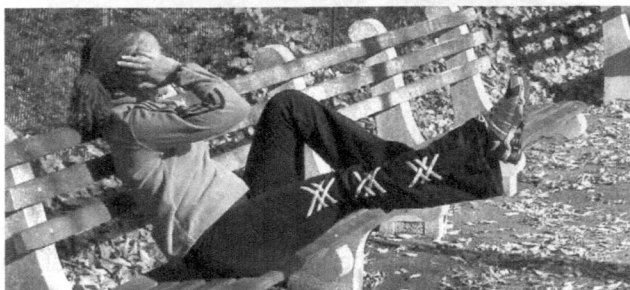

Action
- Sit on the bench, near the edge, and place your hands at the back or side of your head.
- Lean back until your back almost touches the bench.
- Bring one knee up towards the opposite elbow, trying to touch it; hold for a few inhales and exhales.
- Switch and bring your other leg to the opposite elbow and hold for a few inhales and exhales.
- Do as many repetitions as you can, alternating legs, pedaling and coasting along as if you were on a bicycle.

Tips

- You may be more comfortable on a bench that has a flat seat, rather than a curved one.
- — Tone it down: Let your foot land on the ground as the other one comes up, or rest your back on the bench.

138

74. Double leg swivel (intense)

This crunch variation combines a bent leg lift with a rotating movement to include the side (oblique) abdominal muscles.

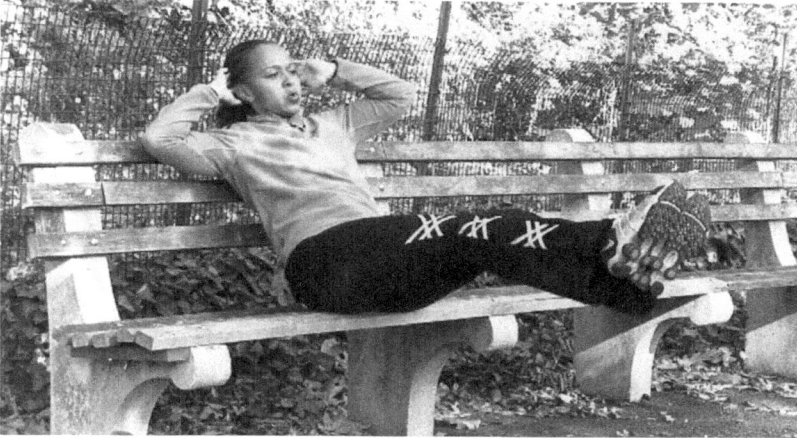

Action

- Sit on the bench, near the edge and place your hands at the back or side of your head.
- Lean back until your back almost touches the bench.
- Bring both knees up towards your chest, trying to touch it.
- Tilt your hips so your knees drop to one side.
- Extend your legs out straight.
- Pull your knees back into your chest as you return your knees and hips to center.
- Tilt your hips so your knees drop to the other side and extend your legs out straight.
- Bend your knees to return to center; continue alternating sides for as many repetitions as you can.

Tips

- You may be more comfortable on a bench that has a flat seat, rather than a curved one.
- — Tone it down: Grab the back of the bench edge with your hands for leverage.

75. Side sit-up (intense)

The bench is your best friend when it comes to positioning your body to target the side muscles (obliques) in this side sit-up.

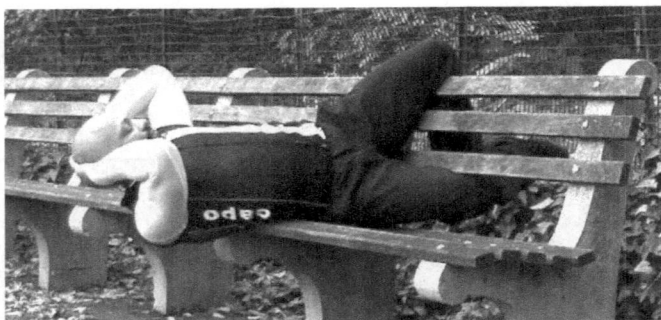

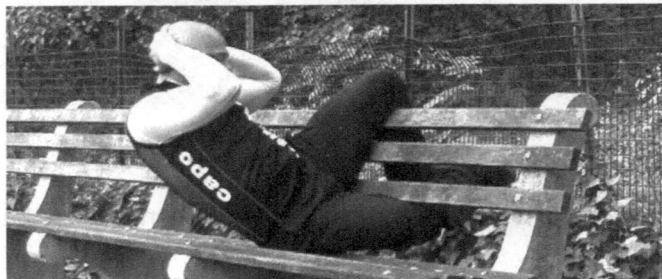

Action

- Lie on the bench on your side, with your body perpendicular to the seat.
- Hook your bottom leg under the bench, between the seat and the back, and the top leg over the top of the back.
- Place your hands behind or at the sides of your head.
- Crunch up, bringing your elbows towards your top knee.
- Do as many repetitions as you can.
- Switch and work the other side.

Tips

- Avoid the temptation to pull or jerk on your head with your hands—very bad for your neck.
- This exercise will be most comfortable if the seat of the bench is flat rather than rounded.

140

76. High-five sit-up (moderate)

You can do this without a partner, but it's so much more fun with a buddy so you get that "high five" feeling. Also, you will be trying to match each other in number of repetitions—a great motivator.

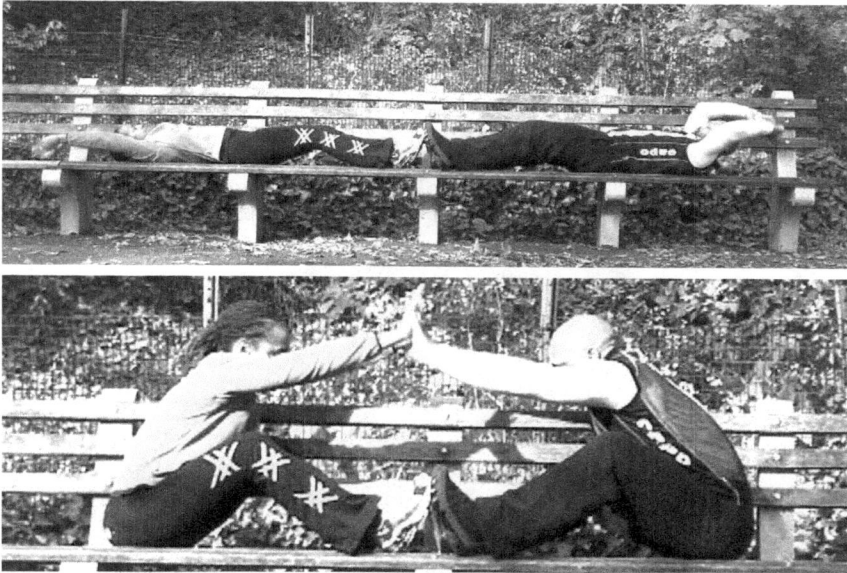

Action

- Lie on the bench with your arms overhead and legs stretched out, your feet touching the bottoms of your partner's feet.
- Contract your abs and lift your shoulder blades and then your back off the bench.
- Come all the way up and forward, and high-five your buddy (or "air-five" if you can't quite reach each other).
- Curl back down and repeat as many times as you can.

Tips

- This will feel most comfortable on a flat seat bench, and one without a back will give you a more spacious feeling.
- If your neck feels strained, support your head with one hand behind it, switching hands with each repetition.
- If you don't have a buddy, aim to touch your toes.

141

77. Leg lift plank (light)

This variation of the plank will work your gluteus muscles in addition to the usual core muscles.

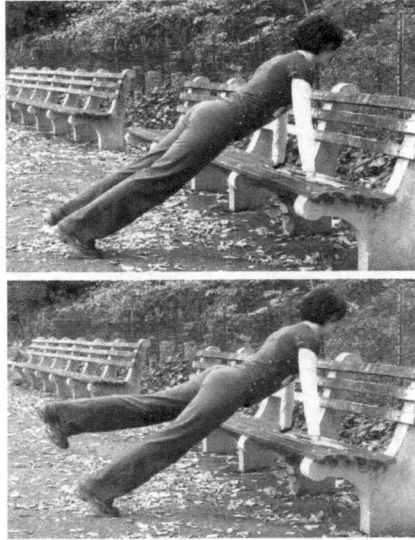

Action

- Standing tall, face the bench and place the palms of your hands on the bench seat, heels up and legs extended long behind you.
- Keep your back flat, with your hips a bit tucked and abdomen contracted, forming a straight line from your feet to your head.
- Raise one leg up until it is on a level with your hips (hips stay level)
- Hold this position for at least one inhale and exhale, keeping the rest of your body firm and in place.
- Switch to your other leg.
- Repeat as many times as you can.

Tips

- This may feel most comfortable on a bench seat that is flat rather than rounded.
- Avoid sinking into your shoulders or letting your hips or head drop down—think of your body as, well, a plank.

+ Take it up a notch: As you raise your left leg, take your right arm up and point to 2 o'clock; as you raise your right leg, take your left arm and point to 10 o'clock.

142

78. Thread the needle (light)

This movement adds a marvelous opening stretch for your chest and shoulder while it works your core muscles. Enjoy!

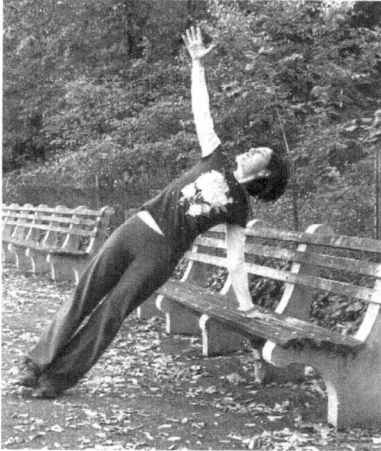

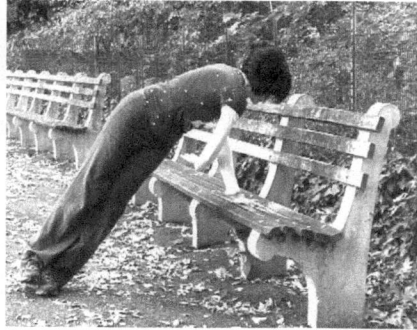

Action

- Standing tall with your side to the bench, place your inside hand on the bench seat, palm down, directly under your shoulder.
- Stack your feet on top of one another or cross one foot in front of the other.
- Contract your core and buttocks and raise your hips so they form a straight line from your feet to your shoulders as you reach up with the outside arm and look up at it.
- Sweep your outside arm out, down, and through the space between your body and the bench ("thread the needle"), twisting your torso but keeping your hips and legs in place.
- Sweep your arm back up and repeat as many times as you can.
- Switch sides and repeat.

Tips

- Avoid sinking into your shoulder and keep your neck long.
- You may find it easier to balance if you look straight ahead rather than at your raised hand.
- **+** Take it up a notch: Balance on your forearm instead of your hand.
- **−** Tone it down: Place your hand on the bench back instead of the seat.

143

CHAPTER FIVE

Endurance

Everyone needs to keep up their cardiovascular system—it's the internal engine that keeps us going. Your heart, lungs, and blood vessels need to work hard every day to stay healthy and in good working order. Endurance exercise, also known as cardiovascular or aerobic exercise, is any exercise that increases your heart rate and breathing for an extended period of time—at least 30 minutes a day— which can be accomplished in three 10-minute segments.

Endurance exercises include high-impact exercises such as boot-camp calisthenics, running or jumping rope; medium-impact workouts such as walking, dancing, or hiking; or low-impact activities such as swimming, bicycling, elliptical machines, stair climbing, and rowing. But let's face it—if you have a history of injuries or a medical condition such as arthritis, long periods of high-impact aerobic exercise are just not in the picture. Even walking long distances may no longer be pleasant. So, for many people, low-impact alternatives are the way to go.

This section has a mixture of low, medium, and high-impact endurance exercises, all using the park bench. Choose whichever is right for you, to augment your other endurance efforts. Throw in some intense moves once you have built up your strength—pushing your body into more intense aerobic activity is what burns more fat, improves your mood, and gives you more energy. Remember too, that most of the strength-building Nancercizes in the other sections will also improve your endurance if you do enough repetitions without resting in between.

You may or may not be preparing to run a 26.2-mile marathon, but we all need to be prepared for the marathon of life. So, make sure that endurance exercises are part of your Nancercize program.

79. Slow march (light)

This exercise is a gentler, low-impact version of mountain climbers, that great standby of boot camp and military style workouts. While mountain climbers are effective, they can be hard on the joints. Here's how to get the benefits without the pain.

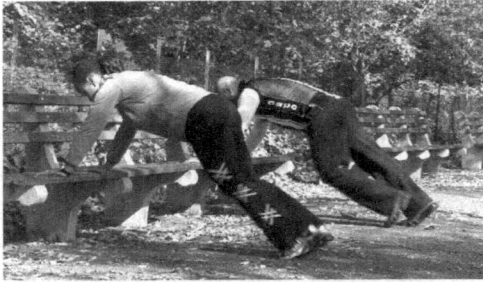

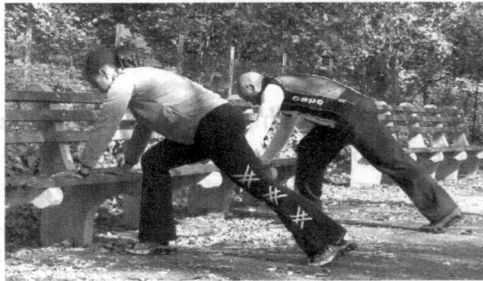

Action
- Stand tall, facing the bench. Place your hands on the bench seat, shoulder-width apart; be on your toes with heels raised, feet about 3 feet from the bench.
- Take a big step towards the bench and then immediately step the foot back away from the bench.
- Repeat with the other foot.
- Repeat as many times as you can, alternating feet, keeping your back and neck elongated.

Tips

➕ Take it up a notch: Pick up the pace and alternate feet by jumping rather than by taking a step in between.

➖ Tone it down: Place your hands on the bench edge (one with a rounded top edge feels most comfortable), or take several small steps.

146

80. Helicopter kick (intense)

This medium-impact exercise was inspired by a move in the Brazilian martial art of capoeira, This type of roundhouse kick is called a *passape* (pah-sah-pay), which in a class or performance is usually performed over the crouching body of your partner.

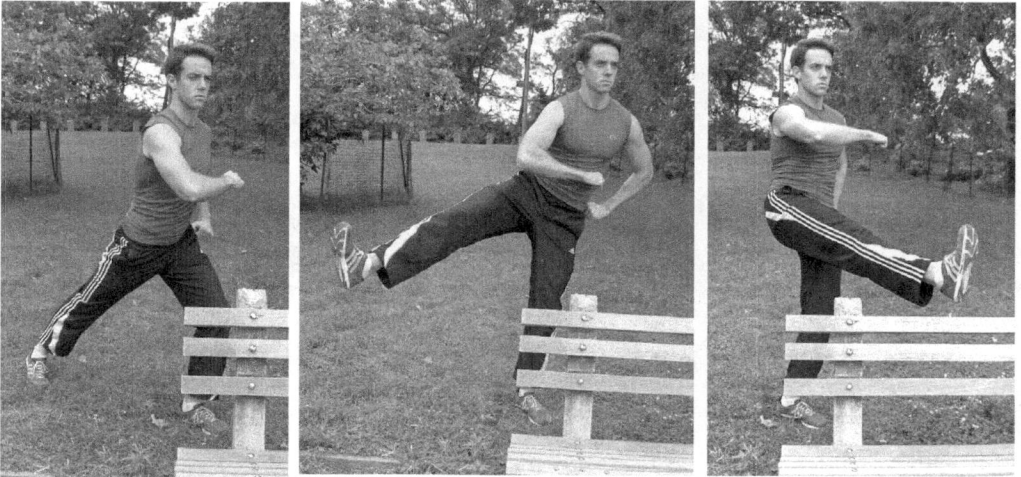

Action

- Stand behind one end of the bench, with your outside foot way back behind you with the leg straight, the leg in front slightly bent.
- Straighten your front leg as you lift the back leg high and sweep it out and over the bench back, landing the foot behind you where it started.
- Repeat as many times as you can on one side.
- Go to the other end of the bench and repeat with the other leg.

Tips

- Helicopter your arms too, to give you balance and momentum.

+ To take it up a notch: Try this circling your leg in the opposite direction (in capoeira that move is called *quiexada* (kay-sha-da).

— Tone it down: Stand in front of the bench and swing your foot over the seat rather than the back.

81. Spider crawl (moderate)

This takes some coordination, but it's so much fun—especially in a group—it's worth it. Once you've got the sequence and feel the rhythm of this low-impact movement, you can get up to quite a speed.

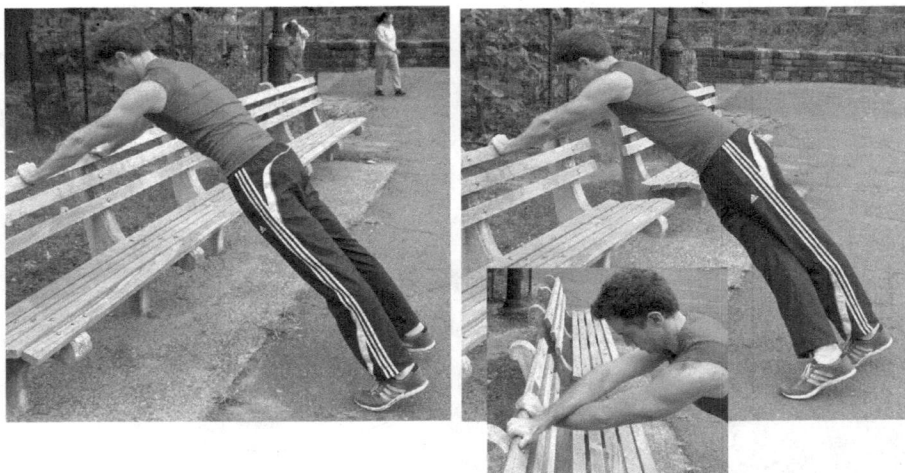

Action

- Stand at one end of the bench, your hands on the back, shoulder-width apart, feet hip-widthapart. Decide which direction you will be traveling—let's start with going to the left.
- Cross your right foot in front of your left; cross your right hand over the left.
- Take a step to the left with your left foot and left hand, uncrossing them.
- Repeat, in a crawling motion, until you get to the end of the bench.
- Reverse direction and repeat as many times as you can.

Tips

- Keep up good form as you travel—back straight, shoulders down, hips even.

➕ Take it up a notch: Crawl your hands along the bench seat instead of the back edge. Gradually increase your speed—see how fast you can Spider crawl.

➖ Tone it down: instead of crossing your hands and feet, just do a step apart followed by a step together to cover the distance.

82. Squat thrust (intense)

For some mysterious (to me) reason this is also called a "burpee"—
maybe if you do them after a meal they make you burp? Anyway, this is a
classic high-impact military and boot camp exercise. A lot of people find
them too difficult when they try them the standard way with hands on the
ground. The thing is, it's really effective, so aren't we lucky we have the
bench alternative, which makes them do-able for more of us?

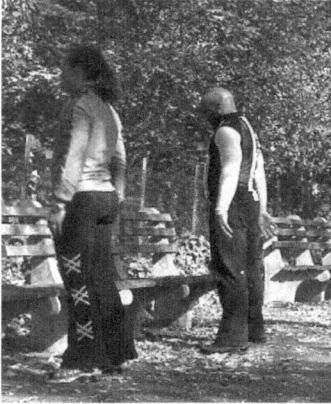

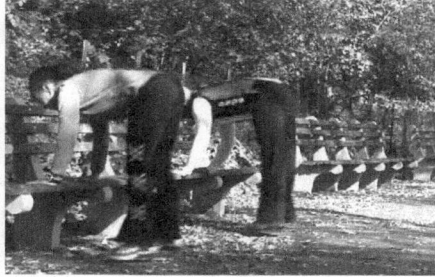

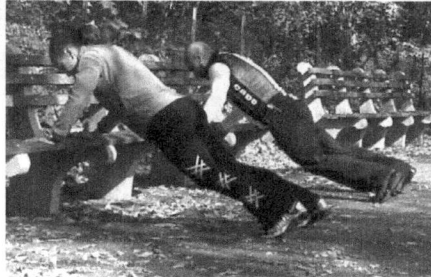

Action
- Stand tall, facing the bench with feet about hip-width apart.
- Place your hands on the bench seat in front of you and squat down as
  you explosively jump your feet out behind you, landing in a push-up
  position.
- Immediately jump your feet again to the starting position and stand up.
- Repeat as many times as you can.

Tips

- Make sure your body is in a straight line when you hit the push-up
  position.
- ➕ Take it up a notch: Add a jump in place with hands overhead, each
  time you jump to the starting position.

83. Hooray step-up (intense)

This is a classic low/moderate-impact step class maneuver, boosted in intensity by the height of the bench.

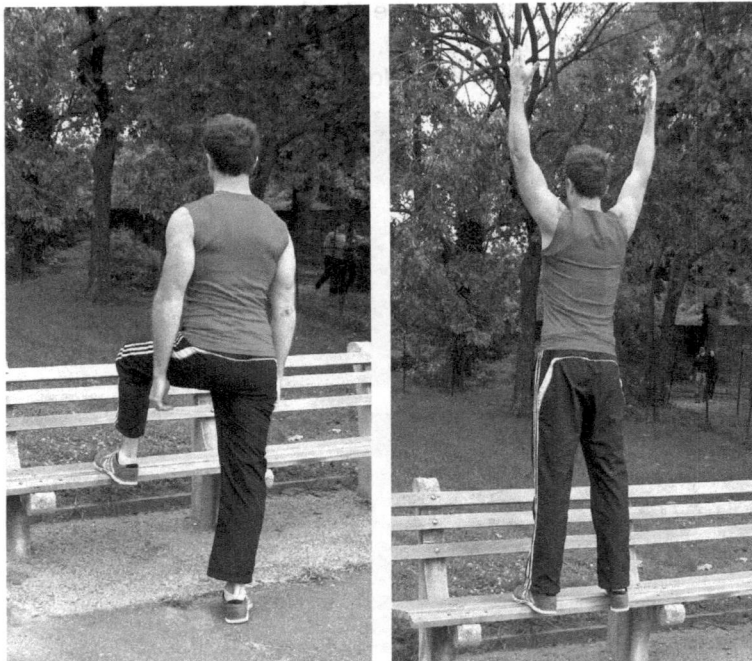

Action

- Stand tall, facing the bench, feet about shoulder-width apart.
- Step up on the bench with one foot.
- Step up with the other foot as you raise your arms overhead.
- Step down on the ground with the starting foot. Step down with the other foot as you lower your arms.
- Repeat as many times as you can, and then use your other leg as the starting leg.

Tips

- Try to step down on your foot lightly with a bent knee to keep this low- to moderate-impact.
- Tone it down: Do this on the ground or on a low curb or step.

84. Tuck jump (intense)

I don't think any other exercise matches this one for sheer simplicity, effectiveness and exuberance. It's got it all! I dare you not to grin and say, "Whee!"

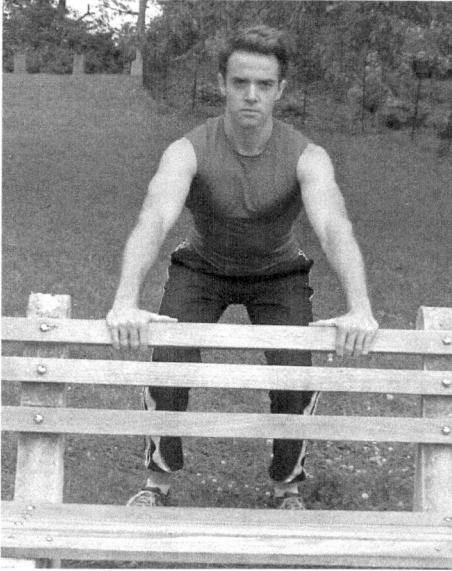

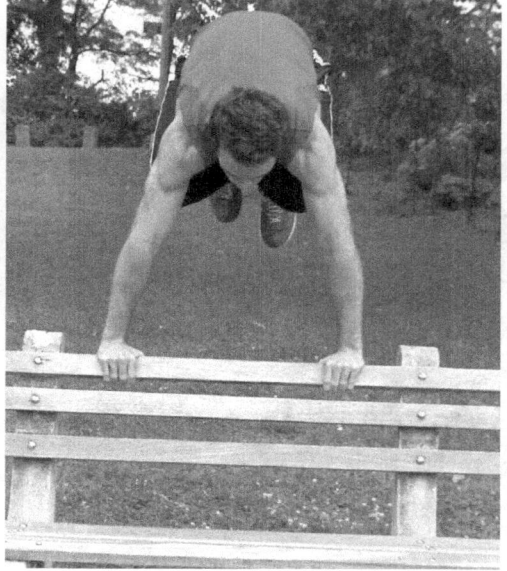

Action
- Stand tall behind the bench, feet together, looking straight ahead.
- Place your hands on the bench back about shoulder-width apart.
- Bend both knees and explosively and joyfully jump as high as you can, tucking your knees and feet under your torso.
- Repeat as many times as you can.

Tips

- Although this can be intense if you jump high for many repetitions, almost anyone can manage a little leap—just keep progressing by making gradually higher and higher jumps and increasing the count.
- Keep knees and feet together during the jump.
- Aim for a soft, bent-knee landing.
- ➕ Take it up a notch: Kick your legs out behind you when you're in the air.
- ➖ Tone it down: Just do a little bunny-hop instead of an explosive jump.

151

85. Jump for joy (intense)

Confession: The first time I tried this high-impact jump it was a disaster! But I eventually did manage to click my heels together, and let me tell you—it was an exhilarating feeling. What a confidence booster. Try it!

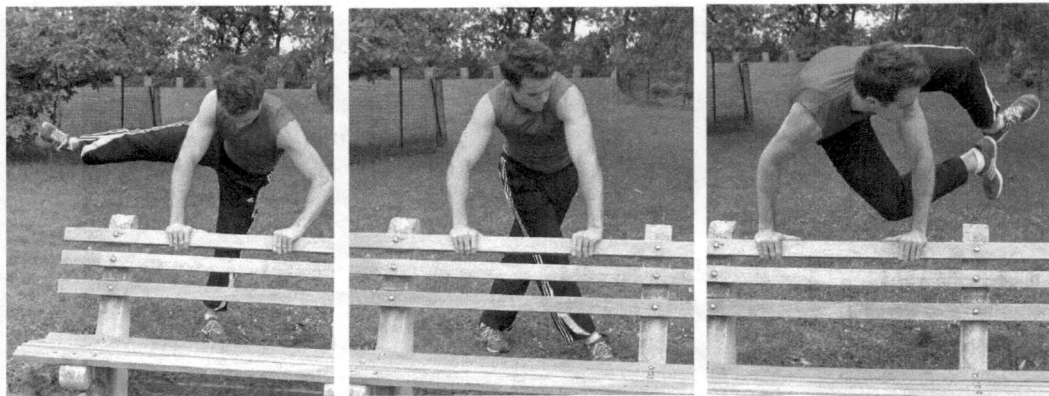

Action
• Let's say you're going to kick to the right. Hold on to the back of the bench and swing your left leg out to the side to start the momentum; bring that leg down, taking a cross step in front of the right leg.
• Bend and straighten both legs as you uncross your legs and explosively jump up to the right, clicking your heels together.
• Land with bent knees and immediately repeat the jump as many times as you can on one side.
• Switch sides and repeat.

Tips

• Use the momentum of the opposite leg to throw both legs up and to the side.
• Be sure to land gently with bent knees to prevent injury with this challenging, high-impact exercise.

86. Dolphin flow (moderate)

Just when you thought you had seen every push-up variation . . . from yoga we get the Dolphin flow. This low-impact move uses the whole body, working wonders for your endurance while strengthening your core and upper body and stretching the back of your legs.

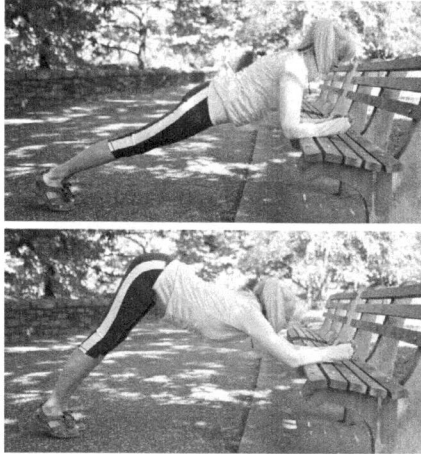

Action
- Start in forearm plank position, with your elbows directly under your shoulders.
- Extend your legs back, toes on the ground and close together.
- Keep your back flat, with your hips a bit tucked and abdomen contracted, your body a straight line from feet to head.
- Engage your abdominals and, pressing with your arms, come into an inverted V position.
- Return to the forearm plank and then the V, alternating positions at least ten times.

Tips

- Keep your head and neck in line with your spine.
- Pull your hips back and up away from the bench to stretch them towards the sky.

➕ Take it up a notch: Press into the bench with your hands and think about reaching your chest towards the ground to activate the stretch.

➖ Tone it down: Bend knees slightly if this makes the stretch more comfortable.

153

CHAPTER SIX

Balance and Flexibility

We take a shower, we cross the street, we change a light bulb in an over-head fixture . . . no big deal. But let me tell you: they *are* a big deal when they become difficult. What these all require is the ability to balance. Bal-ance has become a hot item in the fitness world—gyms are cluttered with balance toys like stability balls, Bosu domes, wedges, wobble boards and so on. But most people don't need such paraphernalia—they need to be able to balance on the ground!

What is balance, anyway? It's simply our ability to stay upright and move through space. Once we're past the wobbly toddler stage, it's something we take for granted. Unbeknownst to us, something called proprioception is hard at work—our body's ability to process the information coming from the soles of our feet, our eyesight, and our inner ears. All these sig-nals pass through our nervous system—our internal "wiring"—to give our bodies a sense of which muscles to activate or deactivate to keep us from falling down.

Unless you've been doing yoga, karate, tai chi, or ballet, you probably haven't been paying attention to preserving or improving your balance. Yet, now you know: balance is one of the key components of fitness. In this section, I include several balance exercises combined with flexibil-ity exercises that are most suitable to do towards the end of your work-out. Flexibility is a key component of balance, as is a strong core. Tight or weak muscles do not help you balance. The beauty of the bench is that it is there to support you when you need it. When your balance im-proves and your core is strong enough, you can try the balance exer-cises in this section (and many of the exercises in the other sections too) without the bench.

Although we might equate poor balance with aging (and it's true that as we age, our balance diminishes), the earlier you start paying attention to balance, the better. It's always easier to maintain good wiring than to re-pair it.

Add five to ten minutes of balance exercises to your workouts three times a week or more. You'll feel steadier, more graceful, and more confident whether you're walking, dancing, or playing competitive sports.

87. Triangle pose (light)

So often I see my students struggling with the balancing aspect of this classic yoga pose. When you use the bench for support, you can concentrate more on your form and relax into the pose, feeling the stretch along your arms and shoulders and in your inner thigh and groin.

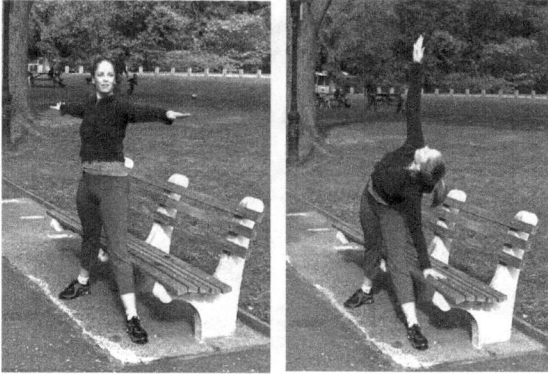

Action
- Stand tall with the back of your legs gently leaning on the edge of the bench for support.
- Separate your feet slightly farther than shoulder-width apart, toes pointing in the direction you will be bending.
- Raise your arms straight out to your sides, palms facing down.
- Bend at your waist, bringing the palm of your hand to the bench seat, and the other arm straight up. Look up at your raised hand.
- Hold for a few inhales and exhales.
- Return to starting position, take a deep breath, and repeat on the other side.
- Reach, reach, reach with your raised arm and your head to feel the stretch fully.

Tips

➕ To tone it down: If you have trouble balancing, look down or straight ahead.
➖ Take it up a notch: Move your supporting hand off the bench and onto your calf, ankle, foot or even the ground.

157

88. Elevated side lunge (moderate)

Like many things in life, this looks so simple, yet, oh how effective and exhilarating it is if you put effort into it! This will help your balance while increasing the flexibility in your inner thighs and hips.

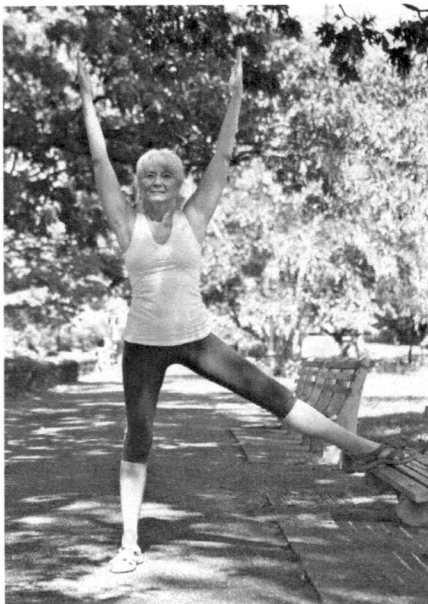

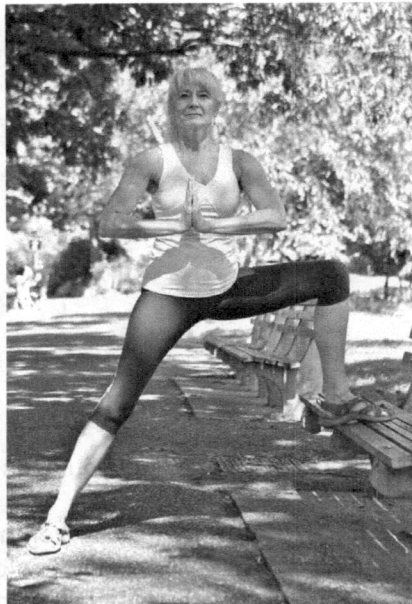

Action

- Stand tall a few feet away from the bench; place your inside leg on the bench seat, foot turned out, and raise both arms overhead.
- Bring the palms of your hands together and lower them to the center of your chest as you bend the knee of the leg that's on the bench.
- Hold for a few inhales and exhales.
- Return to standing, take a breather, and repeat on the other side.
- Reach, reach, reach with your extended arms.

Tips

➕ Take it up a notch: Place your foot on the bench back instead of the seat.

➖ Tone it down: Place your foot on a low curb instead of the bench seat

89. Flying bird (moderate)

I love the simple elegance of this balancing stretch. If you actively reach from fingertips to toes, you'll be elongating your entire body. Feels exhilarating! I imagine this comes close to the way a bird might feel.

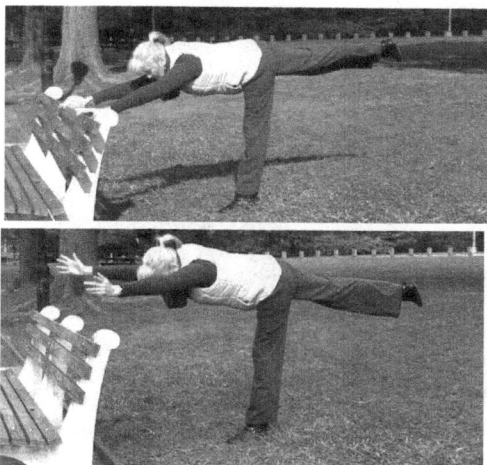

Action
- Stand tall behind the bench, about one arm's distance away from the bench.
- Place both hands on the bench back for support and raise one leg, extending it straight out behind you at hip level.
- Release both hands from the bench and balance for a few inhales and exhales.
- Lower your leg, return to standing, take a breath, and repeat with your other leg.

Tips

- Keep your hips even and your head in line with your spine.
- Gradually increase the time you can balance and hold this position without holding onto the bench.

+ Take it up a notch: Don't hold onto the bench back at all; get into the position and hold it using only your core strength.

90. Gut buster V (intense)

This will work your abs and core while it improves your balance. I often demonstrate this on a stone wall that has a 13-foot drop to the back. This really freaks out my students but is a strong incentive for me to focus!

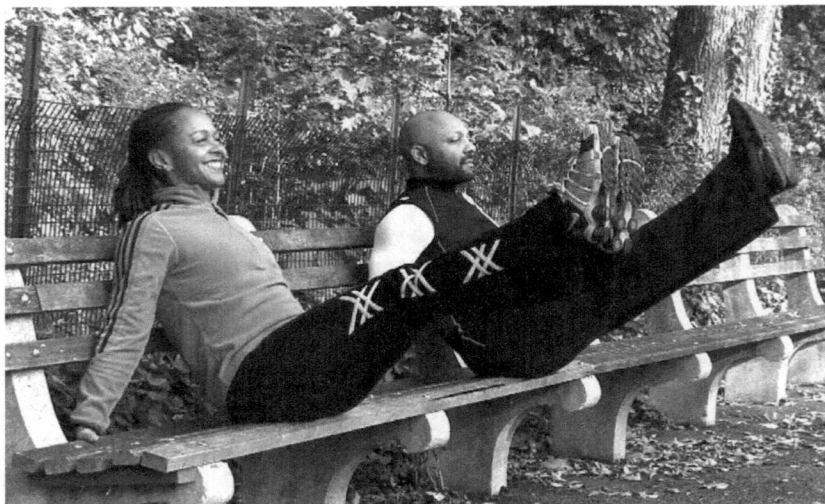

Action
- Sit tall on the edge of the bench, legs glued together, and grab the back edge of the seat with both hands.
- Bend your knees and bring them in towards your chest, then extend them out straight.
- Keep your legs as high and straight as you can, keeping them together, forming a V shape.
- Hold for as long as you can.

Tips

- A bench with a flat seat works better than a rounded seat.
- ➕ Take it up a notch: Let go of the bench and place your hands behind your head or out in front.
- ➖ Tone it down: Hold the position with bent legs and then gradually straighten them as your strength and balance improve.

91. Warrior pose (light)

This classic yoga pose is so much steadier when you have the security of the bench to start with. The warrior helps lengthen your arms, release shoulder tension, and opens up your hips and inner thighs and calves.

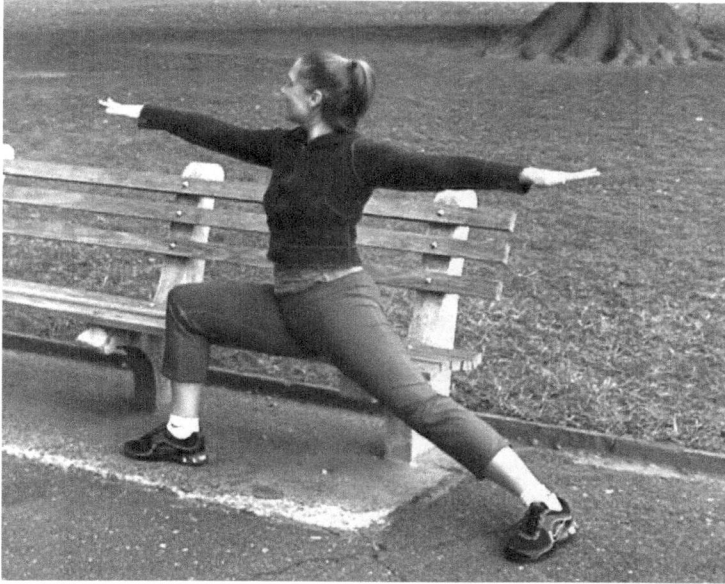

Action
- Stand tall with the back of your legs gently leaning on the edge of the bench for support.
- Separate your feet slightly farther than shoulder-width apart, toes pointing in the direction of the knee you will be bending.
- Raise your arms straight out to your sides, palms facing down.
- Bend your front knee, creating a right angle with your thigh and calf.
- Hold for a few inhales and exhales.
- Return to starting position, take a breath, and repeat on the other side.

Tips

- Avoid letting your bent knee go beyond your toes.
- Think, brave, noble, warrior-like thoughts.

92. Tree pose (moderate)

There's just something so special about doing a tree pose among a bunch of trees. Very inspirational . . . and great for your balance, your core, and your peace of mind.

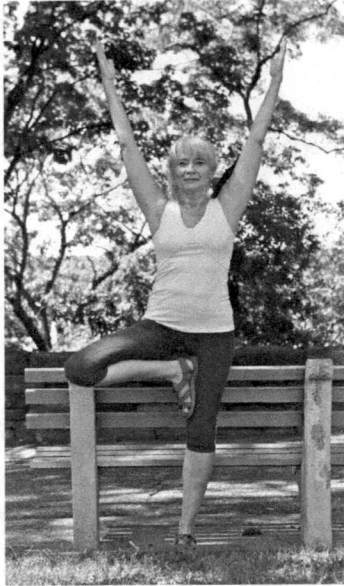

Action
- Stand tall behind the bench, facing away from it, feet touching or a few inches apart.
- Bend one leg, pulling the heel up until the sole rests on the inside of your outer thigh, or as high as it will go.
- Raise both arms over your head and reach for the sky.
- Hold for a few inhales and exhales.
- Release your leg down, take a breath, and repeat with your other leg.

Tips

- Look straight ahead if you can; it helps your balance if you look at something that is stationary, such as a rock on the ground, or another tree in the distance.
- ➕ Take it up a notch: when you're ready, do this without using the bench; try closing your eyes while you balance; wiggle your fingers.

93. Side lunge (light)

This is a nice gentle stretch for your hips and inner thighs. If you're facing a great view—enjoy it!

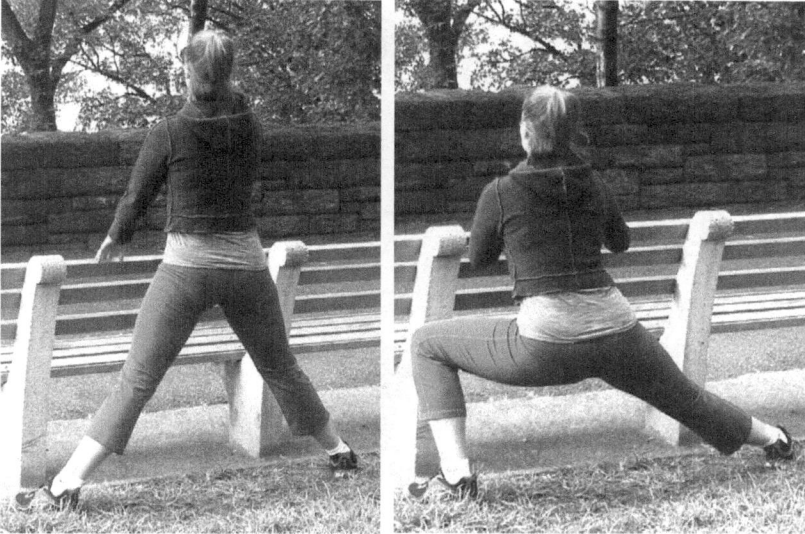

Action

• Stand tall, facing the back of the bench, feet parallel to each other a few feet apart. Rest your hands on the bench back for balance and support.

• Bend one knee, putting your weight back into the heel rather than on the toes.

• Hold for a few inhales and exhales.

• Return to standing, take a breath, and repeat, bending the other leg.

Tips

• Stay tall, elongating through your spine, looking straight ahead of you.

• Be sure that your knee does not extend out past your toes.

94. High lunge (moderate)

Incorporate this stretch into your program and I promise you: your legs and hips will never be the same.

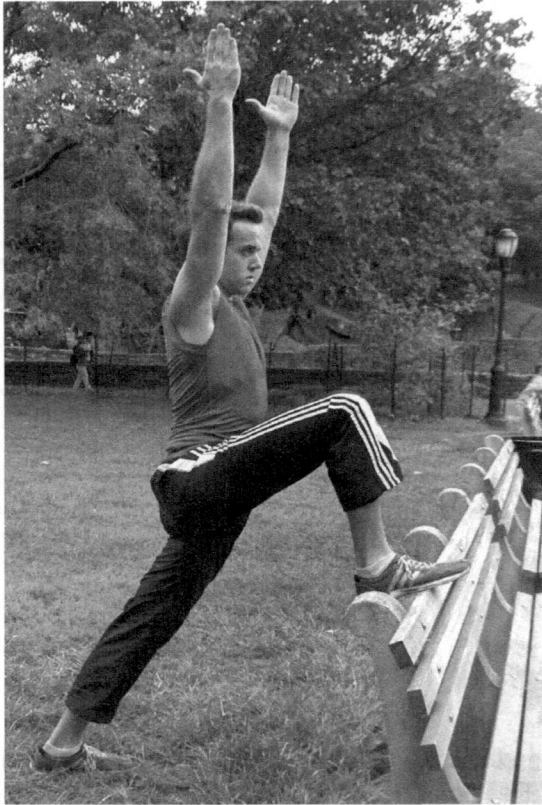

Action
- Stand tall, facing the back of the bench.
- Bring one foot onto the bench back, bending deeply at the knee, letting your body fall towards the bench, while raising your arms all the way up.
- Hold the position for a few inhales and exhales.
- Return to standing position and repeat with your other leg.

Tips

— Take it down a notch: Place your foot on the bench seat rather than the back.

164

95. Flamingo (moderate)

Since flamingos often stand on one leg, I decided to name this balancing stretch after those amazing creatures. In yoga, this is known as dancer's pose or standing bow. When done correctly, this not only works your hips and legs, but opens up your shoulders and chest as well.

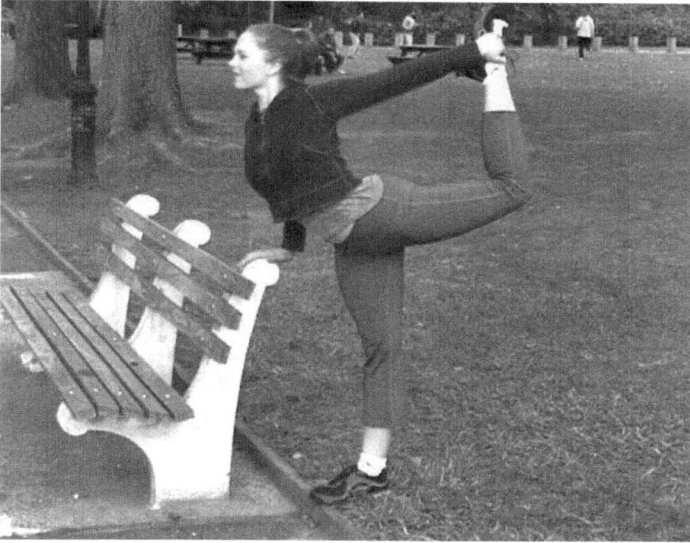

Action

- Stand tall behind the bench with your feet together, one hand resting lightly on the bench back.
- Bend one leg backward, grabbing your foot or ankle with the same side arm.
- Press your foot into your hand for a few inhales and exhales.
- Return to standing, take a breath, and repeat with your other side.

Tips

- Keep your chest high.
- Remember the goal of this exercise is not to press your foot towards your rear, but to stretch it away, pressing against your hand and creating an arch in your back.

➕ Take it up a notch: Let go of the bench and raise your hand upward, reaching towards the sky.

96. Half moon (moderate)

Before I discovered park benches, I would sometimes do this with my back against the wall for stability. The bench works just as well, and being able to place your hand on the seat makes for a gentler version. So, is this a quarter moon?

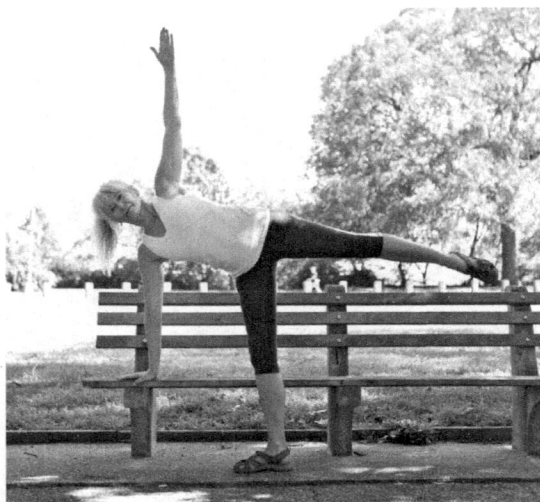

Action
- Stand tall in front of the bench with your feet together, one foot pointed outward, arms at your sides.
- Lift your arms up until they are even with your shoulders in a "T"-shape; bend over sideways from the waist, gently placing one hand on the bench seat so your leg and torso form one straight line, parallel to the ground.
- Hold this pose for a few inhales and exhales.
- Return to standing, take a breath, and repeat in the other direction.
- Reach, reach, reach with your outstretched arm and leg, as well as your head, elongating the pose and feeling the full stretch.

Tips

➕ Take it up a notch: Let go of the bench and raise both arms overhead, using your core strength to balance.

➖ Tone it down: Stand behind the bench, facing towards it, with your supporting hand on the bench back.

166

97. Back bend (moderate)

This is the ultimate anti-sitting-in-front-of-the-computer stretch. Because you are resting your hands on the bench, rather than your ankles, it's a less intense version of the traditional yoga camel pose.

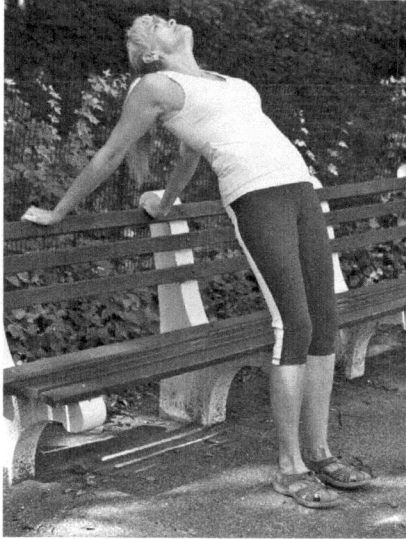

Action
- Stand in front of the bench with your back to it, a few feet away from the seat.
- Reach behind you and place the palms of your hands on the bench back.
- Arch your back and lift your chest and hips high.
- Hold for a few inhales and exhales and then slowly come out of the back bend.
- You can drop your head backward or keep it in line with your spine, whatever is comfortable.

Tips

➕ Take it up a notch: Place your palms on the bench seat instead of the back.

➖ Tone it down: Arch your back less; you'll still feel a nice shoulder and chest stretch.

98. Heavenly stretch (intense)

Even the first half of this stretch feels wonderful. Take your time to reach and settle in to the full extension, which opens up your shoulders, chest, back and entire front of your body like nothing else.

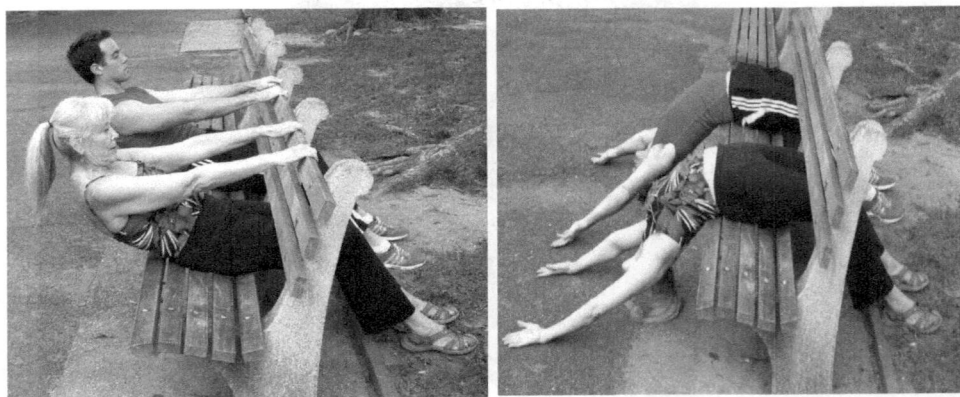

Action
- Sit on the bench, facing the back, and thread your legs though the space between the seat and the back.
- Hold onto the bench back as you start to curl your back down onto the bench and beyond, squeezing your belly button towards your spine and using your core muscles to control the action.
- Raise your arms above your head and let them rest on the ground.
- Hold for a few inhales and exhales.
- Slowly curl up, using your core muscles to control the movement.

Tips

- Strongly engage your abdominal muscles on the way down and up to keep the movement smooth, not jerky.
- — Tone it down: Do just the first part of the stretch, keeping hold of the bench back and pulling your upper back away from the bench.

99. Crossover hip stretch (light)

This is a lovely relaxing position that reaches deep into the hip joint. There's a standing version that works your balance too . . . can you imagine what it looks like? (Hint: Your hands are not clasped under your thigh.)

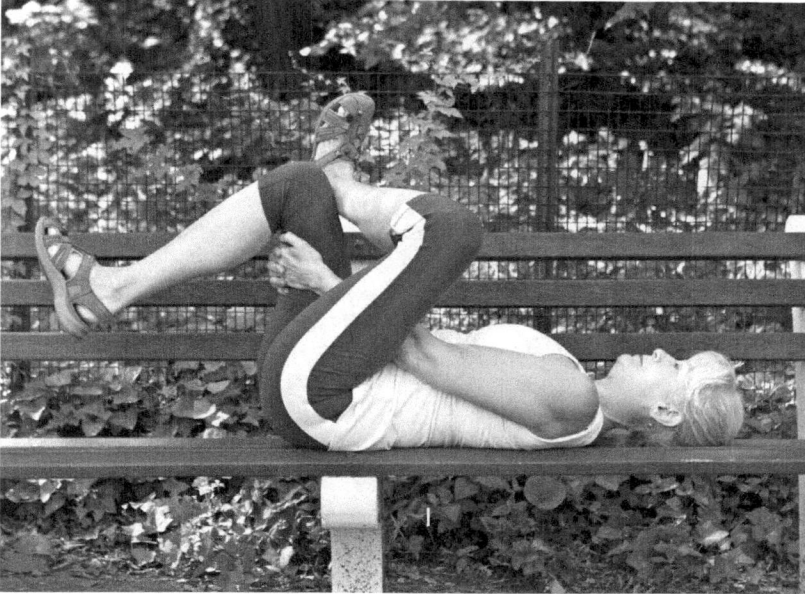

Action

- Lie on your back on the bench, feet flat on the seat and knees bent.
- Cross one foot over the other knee.
- Clasp your hands under the bottom thigh and gently pull the leg towards your chest, keeping your upper body relaxed on the bench.
- Hold for a few inhales and exhales.
- Return to staring position and repeat with your other side.

Tips

- Keep your back long, contracting your abs—don't let your lower back pop up off the bench.

169

100. Seated salute to the sun (light)

Whether the sun is rising, setting, or hiding behind clouds, this is a peaceful way to start or end your day or your workout and re-set your mind and body. It doesn't matter what your level of fitness—I recommend that you incorporate this flowing, relaxing series of movements into your life. Although it is gentle and even meditative in nature, especially if you move slowly, you might also try repeating the series several times at a brisk pace. I once took a yoga class where we performed one hundred full Sun Salutes without stopping!

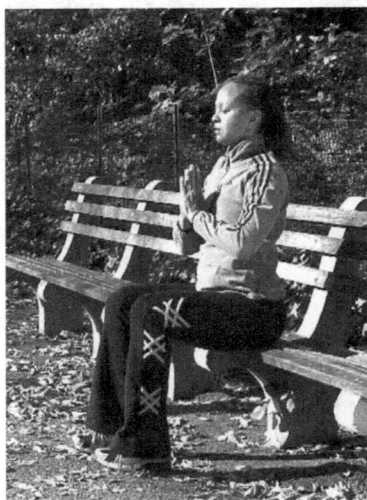

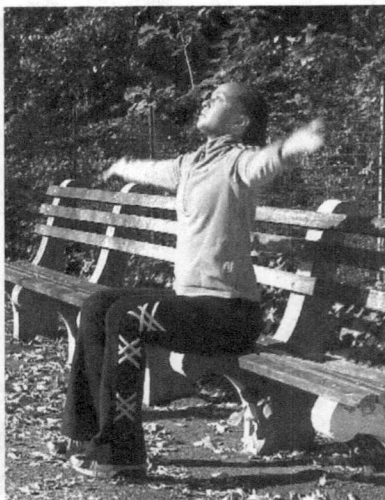

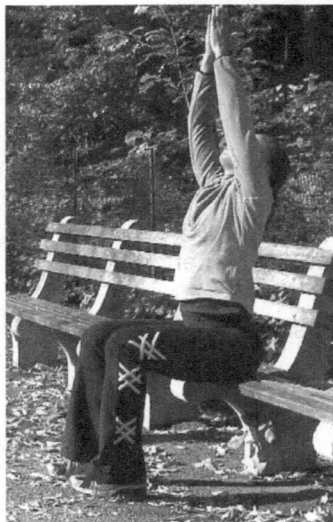

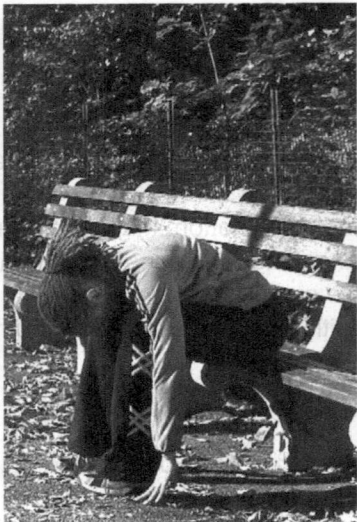

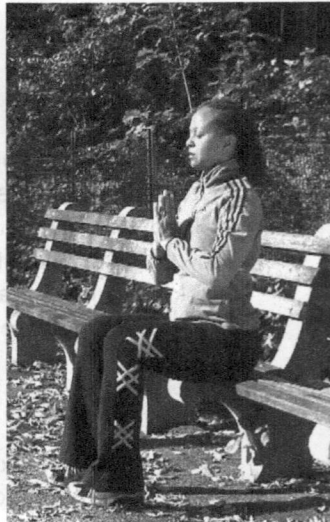

Action

- Sit tall on the edge of the bench, feet flat on the ground directly under your knees, hip-width apart.
- Place your hands in front of your chest, palms together.
- Inhale and sweep your arms out to the sides.
- Continue the sweeping movement up towards the sky, ending with palms together overhead.
- Exhale and sweep your arms outward and downward as you fold your torso over your thighs, resting your fingers on the ground or your ankles.
- Inhale as you sweep your arms out and up again as you roll up your spine, one vertebra at a time, letting your shoulders, neck, and head be the last thing to come into place.
- Bring your hands down, placing them in front of your chest, palms together.
- Repeat as many times as you like.

Tips

- This is most comfortable on a flat seat bench.
- Hold the folded-over position for several inhales and exhales for extra relaxation.
- Try this series with your eyes closed. Listen to the natural sounds around you.

101. Play!

- Now that I've given you 100 ways to use a park bench to get stronger and more flexible, to increase your endurance and improve your balance—it's your turn to play.
- What's fitness for, except to help us enjoy life?
- Now's your moment to be creative. Use your imagination to invent your own Nancercizes—the sky's the limit, and you don't have to play alone!

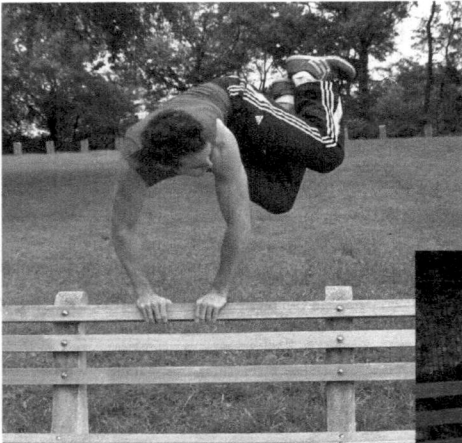

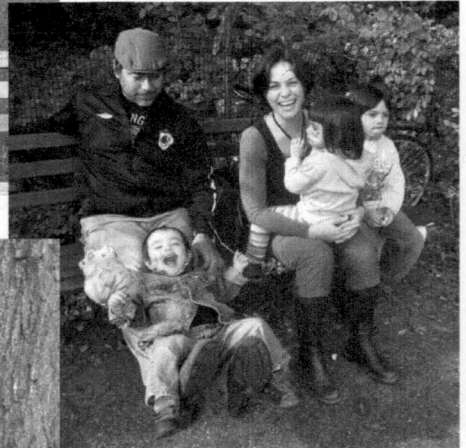

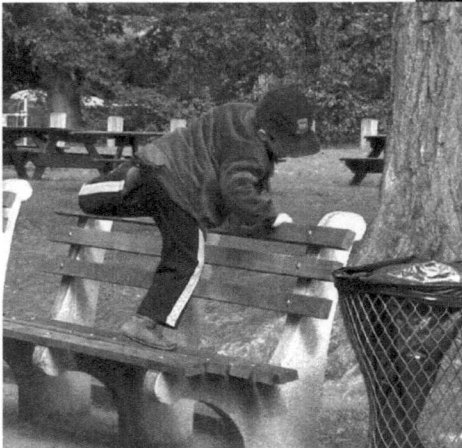

Part III

The Workouts

36 Workouts for Every Occasion and Level of Fitness

What follows are 12 workouts for each of the three levels of intensity—for a total of 36 workouts. These workouts range from a full 60-minute workout to a tiny but powerful 5-minute break, with everything in between. It doesn't matter how little or how much time you have—you'll find something to get your circulation going.

When following the workouts, bear in mind that the time spans for the segments of the workouts are estimates; if you want to spend longer on one particular exercise, do that, within the guidelines. If you need less time, take less. For the aerobic segments, I've specified walking, jogging, and running . . . but by all means use whatever form of aerobic exercise you like, from stair climbing to rebounding, depending on your outdoor "gym."

Do the workouts as is, or vary them by choosing different exercises in the same category. Realize that you may not be able to work out at the same level across all categories. For example, you might be able to do high intensity push-ups, but if you lack flexibility start with the light version of a flexibility exercise. The opposite can hold true—you may be quite flexible but lack muscle strength. So, in any given workout use the exercises from the column appropriate for you in the various categories. For instance, if you do the 60-minute workout, you might do the exercises in the light column for flexibility, the intense column for lower body strength, and moderate column for upper body strength, and so on. Also, since most exercises have a total of three versions, use the version of the exercise that is appropriate to your level—you may want to take it up a notch (+) or tone it down (-). Always listen to your body!

For another form of variety, don't hesitate to mix them up during the day or during the week. For example, you might have four 5-minute breaks during the day, or two 15-minute time slots on one day, or a full hour another day. In whatever way you adapt the workouts to your particular needs, I guarantee you'll never be bored or at a loss for ideas or time.

The workouts are:

- Classic 60-Minute Total Body Nancercize Circuit
- Classic 30-Minute Total Body Nancercize Circuit
- 23-Minute Fat Burner
- 20-Minute Lower Body Workout
- 20-Minute Core Workout
- 20-Minute Upper Body Workout
- 20-Minute Stress Buster
- 15-Minute Lunchtime Quickie
- 15-Minute Energizer
- 10-Minute Mini-Mix
- 10-Minute Spa Vacation
- 5-Minute Emergency Break

If you'd like to see more workout ideas, visit my website nancercize.net and subscribe to my newsletter. If you have questions, email me at questions@nancercize.net.

Classic 60-Minute Total Body Nancercize Circuit

That's right: the highlight of your day!

Time in minutes	Category	Light	Moderate	Intense
5	**Warm up** **Flexibility** (10-30 seconds each, repeat sequence)	Walk 1. Side stretch 2. Table top stretch 9. Seated twist 11. Triceps stretch 12. Seated chair	Walk 3. Downward facing dog 6. Crossover stretch 8. Knee to nose 10. Seated eagle 15. Flowing lunge	Walk 7. Flowing hamstring stretch 13. See-saw 17. Crescent stretch 18. Butterfly stretch 20. Forward flow and twist
10	**Aerobic**	Brisk walk	Jog	Run
5	**Lower body** (Total of 1 minute each, with short break in between)	22. Hamstring curl (-) 27. Back leg lift 28. Side leg lift 29. Front leg lift 31. Up on your toes	22. Hamstring curl 23. Standing donkey side kick 24. Leg circles 25. Hover squat 26. Stomp on the brake	38. Sky kick 39. Xtreme knee lift 40. Split squat 41. Power jump 42. Power tap
10	**Aerobic**	Brisk walk	Jog	Run
5	**Upper body** (Total of 1 minute each, with short break in between)	44. Modified push up 47. Walking push up (-) 52. Basic dip (toned down) 50. Walk the plank 51. Leg lift push up	45. Pulsing push up 47. Walking push up 53. Cross legged dip 48. Push off and clap 49. Side plank and arm circle	55. One arm tricep push up 56. Power push up 57. One arm power push up 58. Handstand push up 59. Wheelbarrow
10	**Aerobic**	Brisk walk	Jog	Run
5	**Core** (Total of 1 minute each, with short break in between)	60. Basic sit up (-) 63. Basic bicycle (-) 64. Modified plank 72. Air pump 77. Leg lift plank	60. Basic sit up 61. Hug yourself and twist 62. Hippy dippy plank 63. Basic bicycle 68. Roll up	63. Basic bicycle (+) 65. Double leg lift 66. Scissors kick 67. Flutter kick 72. Air pump (+)

Classic 30-Minute Total Body Nancercize Circuit

There's no better way to spend a half hour.

Time in minutes	Category	Light	Moderate	Intense
2	**Warm up**	Walk	Walk	Walk
2	**Lower body** (Total of 1 minute each, with short break in between)	22. Hamstring curl (-) 28. Side leg lift	30. Static squat 34. L kick	38. Sky kick 39. Power jump
10	**Aerobic**	Brisk walk	Jog	Run
2	**Upper body** (Total of 1 minute each, with short break in between)	44. Modified push up 52. Basic dip (-)	45. Pulsing push up 54. One-legged dip	56. Power push up 53. Cross-legged dip (+)
10	**Aerobic**	Brisk walk	Jog	Run
2	**Core** (Total of 1 minute each, with short break in between)	60. Basic sit up (-) 64. Modified plank	69. Hip lift 70. Elbow plank	63. Basic bicycle (+) 71. Double leg swivel
2	**Balance and Flex** (10-30 seconds each, repeat sequence)	87. Triangle 100. Seated salute to the sun	96. Half moon 97. Back bend	92. Tree (+) 98. Heavenly stretch

23-Minute Fat Burner

Take advantage of a modified high intensity interval training (HIIT) technique.

Time in minutes	Category	Light	Moderate	Intense
1	**Warm up**	Walk	Walk	Walk
1	**Lower Body**	27. Back leg lift	26. Stomp on the brake	38. Sky kick
4	**Aerobic** (alternating) (1 minute each)	Walk/Brisk walk	Jog/Run	Run/Sprint
1	**Core**	72. Air pump	69. Hip lift	74. Double leg swivel
4	**Aerobic** (alternating) (1 minute each)	Walk/Brisk walk	Jog/Run	Run/Sprint
1	**Upper Body**	44. Modified push up	45. Pulsing push up	56. Power push up
4	**Aerobic** (alternating) (1 minute each)	Walk/Brisk walk	Jog/Run	Run/Sprint
1	**Lower Body**	28. Side leg lift	23. Standing donkey side kick	41. Power jump
4	**Endurance** (Total of 1 minute each, with short break in between)	79. Slow march 83. Hooray step up (-) 89. Slow march 81. Spider crawl (-)	80. Helicopter kick, clockwise (-) 84. Jump for joy (-) 80. Helicopter kick, counterclockwise (-) 86. Dolphin flow	82. Squat thrust 83. Hooray step up 84. Tuck jump 85. Jump for joy
1	**Lower Body**	29. Front leg lift	35. Basic squat	43. One-legged squat
1	**Balance and Flex**	93. Side lunge	95. Flamingo	94. High lunge

177

20-Minute Lower Body Workout
Because your buns WANT to be made of steel.

Time in minutes	Category	Light	Moderate	Intense
1	**Warm up**	Walk	Walk	Walk
10	**Aerobic**	Brisk walk	Jog	Run
6	**Lower body** (Total of 1 minute each, with short break in between)	22. Hamstring curl (-) 27. Back leg lift 28. Side leg lift 29. Front leg lift 31. Up on your toes 34. L kick (-)	22. Hamstring curl 23. Standing donkey side kick 24. Leg circles 35. Basic Squat 36. Squat and cross 37. Tuck and kick	38. Sky kick 38. Xtreme knee lift 40. Split squat 41. Power jump 42. Power tap 43. One-legged squat
2	**Flexibility** (30 seconds each, repeat entire sequence)	2. Table top stretch 6. Crossover stretch (-)	3. Downward dog 6. Crossover stretch	7. Flowing hamstring 18. Butterfly
1	**Balance and Flex**	91. Warrior	94. High lunge	88. Elevated side lunge

20-Minute Core Workout

Show your belly who's in charge.

Time in Minutes	Category	Light	Moderate	Intense
1	**Warm up**	Walk	Walk	Walk
10	**Aerobic**	Brisk walk	Jog	Run
6	**Core** (Total of 1 minute each, with short break in between)	64. Modified plank 72. Air pump 77. Leg lift plank 78. Thread the needle 60. Basic sit up (-) 63. Basic bicycle (-)	61. Hug yourself and twist 62. Hippy dippy plank 68. Roll up 70. Elbow plank 73. Coasting bicycle 76. High-five sit up	65. Double leg lift 66. Scissor kick 67. Flutter kick 73. Coasting bicycle (+) 74. Double leg swivel 75. Side sit up
2	**Flexibility** (30 seconds each, repeat entire sequence)	1. Side stretch 3. Downward facing dog	4. Deep squat stretch 19. Upward facing dog	5. Over easy (+) 17. Crescent stretch
1	**Balance and Flex**	97. Back bend (-)	89. Flying bird	98. Heavenly stretch

20-Minute Upper Body Workout
You're on your way to best toned arms in town.

Time in minutes	Category	Light	Moderate	Intense
1	Warm up	Walk	Walk	Walk
10	Aerobic	Brisk walk	Jog	Run
6	Upper body (Total of 1 minute each, with short break in between)	44. Modified push up 47. Walking push up (-) 50. Walk the plank 51. Leg lift push up 52. Basic dip (-)	45. Pulsing push up 47. Walking push up 53. Cross legged dip 48. Push off and clap 49. Side plank and arm circle	55. One arm triceps push up 56. Power push up 57. One arm power push up 58. Handstand push up 59. Wheelbarrow
2	Flexibility (30 seconds each, repeat entire sequence)	11. Triceps stretch 12. Seated chair pose	5. Over easy 10. Seated eagle	7. Flowing hamstring stretch 13. See-saw
1	Balance and Flex	100. Seated salute to the sun	95. Flamingo	97. Back bend (+)

20-Minute Stress Buster

When you feel the urge for fight or flight: Throw your bodyweight around instead.

Time in minutes	Category	Light	Moderate	Intense
1	**Warm up**	Walk	Walk	Walk
2	**Flexibility** (30 seconds each, repeat entire sequence)	1. Side stretch 9. Seated twist	8. Knee to nose 15. Flowing lunge	13. See - saw 21. Wishbone
7	**Aerobic**	Brisk walk	Brisk walk or jog	Brisk walk or run
2	**Flexibility** (30 seconds each, repeat entire sequence)	3. Downward facing dog 4. Deep squat stretch (-)	4. Deep squat stretch 5. Over easy (+)	17. Crescent stretch 20. Forward flow and twist
5	**Endurance** (Total of 1 minute each, with short break in between)	79. Slow march 81. Spider crawl (-) 83. Hooray step up (-) 86. Dolphin flow (-) 89. Slow march	80. Helicopter kick, clockwise (-) 81. Spider crawl 84. Jump for joy (-) 86. Dolphin flow 80. Helicopter kick, counterclockwise (-)	82. Squat thrust 83. Hooray step up 84. Tuck jump 82. Squat 85. Jump for joy
3	**Balance and Flex** (10-30 seconds each, repeat sequence)	87. Triangle pose 91. Warrior 93. Side lunge	89. Flying bird 92. Tree 96. Half moon	94. High lunge 97. Back bend (+) 98. Heavenly stretch

15-Minute Lunchtime Quickie

For your pre-lunch "appetizer." (It will have the opposite effect.)

Time in minutes	Category	Light	Moderate	Intense
1	**Warm up**	Walk	Walk	Walk
1	**Lower body**	35. Basic squat (-)	32. Bridge with leg lift	33. Horizon kick
5	**Aerobic**	Brisk walk	Jog	Run
1	**Upper body**	51. Push up with leg lift	46. Push off	56. Power push up
5	**Endurance** (Total of 1 minute each, with short break in between)	79. Slow march 81. Spider crawl (-) 79. Slow march 86. Dolphin flow (-) 79. Slow march	79. Slow march (+) 80. Helicopter kick (-) 81. Spider crawl 83. Hooray step up (-) 86. Dolphin flow	80. Helicopter kick 82. Squat thrust 83. Hooray step up 84. Tuck jump 85. Jump for joy
1	**Core**	64. Modified plank	71. Knee drop plank	65. Double leg lift
1	**Balance and Flex**	100. Seated salute to the sun	100. Seated salute to the sun	100. Seated salute to the sun

15-Minute Energizer

After this workout you won't even want that candy bar!

Time in minutes	Category	Light	Moderate	Intense
1	**Warm up**	Walk	Walk	Walk
2	**Lower body** (Total of 1 minute each, with short break in between)	27. Back leg lift 28. Side leg lift	23. Standing donkey side kick 26. Stomp on the brake	38. Sky kick 41. Power jump
5	**Aerobic**	Walk	Jog	Run
2	**Core** (Total of 1 minute each, with short break in between)	72. Air pump 77. Thread the needle	69. Hip lift 71. Knee drop plank	74. Double leg swivel 75. Side sit up
4	**Endurance** (Total of 1 minute each, with short break in between)	79. Slow march 83. Hooray step up (-) 89. Slow march 81. Spider crawl (-)	80. Helicopter kick, clockwise (-) 84. Jump for joy (-) 86. Dolphin flow 80. Helicopter kick, counterclockwise (-)	82. Squat thrust 83. Hooray step up 84. Tuck jump 85. Jump for joy
1	**Balance and Flex**	93. Side lunge	95. Flamingo	98. Heavenly stretch

183

15-Minute Lunchtime Quickie

For your pre-lunch "appetizer." (It will have the opposite effect.)

Time in minutes	Category	Light	Moderate	Intense
1	**Warm up**	Walk	Walk	Walk
1	**Lower body**	35. Basic squat (-)	32. Bridge with leg lift	33. Horizon kick
5	**Aerobic**	Brisk walk	Jog	Run
1	**Upper body**	51. Push up with leg lift	46. Push off	56. Power push up
5	**Endurance** (Total of 1 minute each, with short break in between)	79. Slow march 81. Spider crawl (-) 79. Slow march 86. Dolphin flow (-) 79. Slow march	79. Slow march (+) 80. Helicopter kick (-) 81. Spider crawl 83. Hooray step up (-) 86. Dolphin flow	80. Helicopter kick 82. Squat thrust 83. Hooray step up 84. Tuck jump 85. Jump for joy
1	**Core**	64. Modified plank	71. Knee drop plank	65. Double leg lift
1	**Balance and Flex**	100. Seated salute to the sun	100. Seated salute to the sun	100. Seated salute to the sun

10-Minute Mini-Mix

Got 10 minutes? Rinse. Repeat as needed.

Time in minutes	Category	Light	Moderate	Intense
1	**Warm up**	Walk	Walk	Walk
2	**Lower body** (Total of 1 minute each, with short break in between)	28. Side leg lift 30. Static squat (-)	22. Hamstring curl 25. Hover squat	40. Split squat 41. Power jump
2	**Endurance** (Total of 1 minute each, with short break in between)	79. Slow march 81. Spider crawl (-)	83. Hooray step up (-) 86. Dolphin flow	80. Helicopter kick 85. Jump for joy
2	**Core** (Total of 1 minute each, with short break in between)	60. Basic sit up (-) 64. Modified plank	60. Basic sit up 68. Rollup	66. Scissor kick 67. Flutter kick
2	**Endurance** (Total of 1 minute each, with short break in between)	79. Slow march 86. Dolphin flow (-)	80. Helicopter kick (-) 81. Spider crawl	82. Squat thrust 84. Tuck jump
1	**Balance and Flex**	91. Warrior pose	89. Flying bird	98. Heavenly stretch

5-Minute Emergency Break

The next best thing to a nap.

Time in minutes	Category	Light	Moderate	Intense
1	Warm up	Walk	Walk	Walk
1	Lower body	35. Basic squat (-)	35. Basic squat	40. Split squat
1	Endurance	79. Slow march	86. Dolphin flow	84. Tuck jump
1	Core	72. Air pump	63. Basic bicycle	65. Double leg swivel
1	Balance and Flex	100. Seated salute to the sun	95. Flamingo	92. Tree (+)

Nancercize

Author's Afterword

Author's Afterword

Recently a philanthropist offered to donate expensive outdoor exercise equipment to a New York City park, to be specifically to be used by the seniors who exercised in the park. What was so interesting, and what made news, was that the seniors declined the generous offer with an appreciative but definite "'No thanks!'" They made it clear that they preferred to go to classes with a real live instructor, using just the equipment that the park already had. They wanted to have the money spent on an experienced person to motivate and lead them, and they definitely wanted to be part of a group. Even with the fanciest equipment, they didn't want to exercise on their own.

I find this both inspiring and instructive, because that, of course, is what Nancercize is all about. I am also excited to see how many fitness trainers, both established and beginners alike, are adopting the principles of the Nancercize program. They are committed to using outdoor exercise to likewise bring their current and future clients to a heightened state of health and happiness, working singly and in groups on Mother's Nature's beautiful grounds and under her open skies!

The desire that these people expressed— to follow a leader and to be part of a group that is aligned in purpose and going in the same direction— leads me to another story. I actually found this narrative, which is also a kind of morality tale, in a three-minute video called "Pulling Together." It is immensely moving, and you can click on this link http://www.pullingtogethermovie.com/to view it for yourself.

This video tells the story of migrating geese, and how they are able to fly vast distances as a group, 71% farther than if any one goose were to fly alone. They can achieve this amazing feat in tandem because they have a common purpose and a sense of community. Flying in V-formation, they create an uplift updraft, which helps the birds behind them. They also take turns leading to give each other a rest. When one of the group is too weak or injured to keep flying, two other geese accompany the sick goose to the ground and stay with him or her until that goose either can return to formation or dies. Then the two return to the flock to avoid the drag and resistance of flying alone, or form a new group of their own. Best of all, they honk to encourage those up front.

Author's Afterword

The statistics tell their own tale: Antidepressants are now the most pre-scribed drugs in the US. Over two-thirds of Americans are overweight or obese, and more than one-third of our children and teens are likewise overweight or obese. In excess of 300,000 people die each year from diseases and health conditions related to a sedentary lifestyle and poor eating habits, nearly as many as the number who die from smoking. In fi-nancial terms, we as a nation spend a whopping $117 billion annually treating conditions related to overweight and obesity. How frightening is this: There are realistic predictions that unless we can reverse this trend, diabetes—which can lead to blindness, kidney failure, heart disease and other serious consequences—will strike one out of three of the children who were born in 2000 and beyond.

We can write a better story by becoming more active.

The real key to success is to invite others to Nancercize with you. My se-cret goal (shhh!) is to train people like you to start up your own little group, even if it's just a group of two or three. Bring your friends and fam-ily to the park. Connect with nature. Connect with the earth. As a side benefit you'll find you're also enhancing your connection with each other!

One more thing in the connection arena: I would like you to connect with your real power, even as one individual. Make your voice heard, just as those seniors did, to make sure that we build more neighborhood parks, that those parks have plenty of fitness-friendly benches, and that funds are used to hire Nancercize instructors to spread the word. And, if you can, contribute to nonprofit organizations that promote outdoor physical activity.

If you're at all concerned about the environment, become an advocate for Nancercize (after you experience it for yourself, of course). It's simply the most eco-friendly form of exercise there is, because it requires no extra equipment and no fuel except human power.

In the beginning of this book I talked about how ending our exercise group brought tears to the eyes of the fifty people who were part of that group. They were sad at the thought of losing something we had created together, something that had changed all our lives for the better.

Are you ready to make your life and the lives of those you care about happier, healthier, and richer in all of the ways that truly count? Then please accept my invitation to do it . . . ...

Outside!

In a park!

Together!

With a partner or in a group!

On a bench!

Dancing with life . . .

The Nancercize way

Credits

Nancercize Instructors/Fitness Models

This book would not exist without the photos of the exercises being demonstrated by these fabulous fitness instructors.

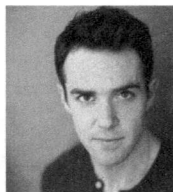

Charles Andrew Callaghan, A.C.E, is a personal trainer at Clay Health Club + Spa in New York City. Whenever possible, he trains his clients outdoors, in the fresh air where exercise just feels natural. Charles is a trapeze artist and an amateur cyclist with a keen interest in "Fitness for a Cause" including the California Livestrong Challenge for Cancer Research. Chad is also an actor and graduate of Yale University and the National Theater Conservatory. www.charlesandrewcallaghan.com

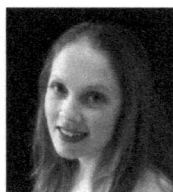

Shawna Emerick, R.Y.T., has been teaching yoga for over seven years. she holds two 200-hour Yoga Teaching Certificates as well as many other continuing education teaching hours in Pre-natal and children's Yoga. Shawna also runs her modern dance company, Vital Dance, offers Thai Yoga, and practices Reiki. She teaches free yoga classes in Fort Tryon Park and believes that one of the best places to do yoga and dance is outdoors—the joy of moving and feeling as big and wide as the sky itself can give everyone the energy to motivate, connect, and become creative while feeling healthy! www.ShawnaYoga.com

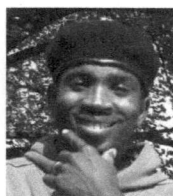

Donovan Green, A.C.E., a leading expert in Fitness and Self-Defense, is the personal trainer to Dr. Mehmet Oz. His winning personality gets people moving with high energy and pure understanding of proper body mechanics. he has appeared in numerous published articles and on public broadcasts and published articles such as the Dr. Oz show, Hot 97, and Oprah Radio. His exciting and high-energy fitness program called *Extreme Defensive Fitness* (EDF) is often performed outdoors. EDF is a self-defense program designed to educate men, women, and children on ways to defend themselves while getting an awesome workout that is fun, challenging, and stress-relieving. http://www.extremedefensivefitness.com/

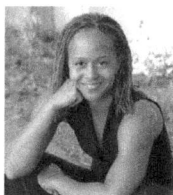

Lisa Priestly, CPT, RYT-200, HLC, began in sales and communication skills training but over the last fifteen years she found her passion and shifted her career into the health and fitness industry. Today she is a Certified Personal Trainer, a Registered Yoga Teacher and Holistic Lifestyle Coach. Her integrated approach to vital living is highlighted in her book, Stepping Stones to Success. Lisa walks her talk, with a daily meditation and yoga practice, as well as teaching free yoga classes in Fort Tryon Park. She was the first African-American woman to complete the bike Race Across America in 2010. Lisa believes that exercise should not be limited by location. There is *always* a possibility and no excuses for not exercising.

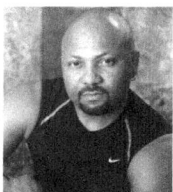

Roderick "Priest" Priestly, CPT, HLC II, is known by his peers and clients as a mentor, role model, and coach. Priest has been the catalyst for change in the lives of many during his twenty-plus years of teaching and training. he holds two second-degree black belts, and his integrated martial arts style is based on training in Jeet Kune Do, Jujitsu, Judo and Shotokan Karate. He is a C.H.E.K. Institute Level II Holistic Lifestyle Coach, and holds certifications from the East Coast Alliance and American Council on Exercise. Although he spends much of his time in gyms, health clubs, and fitness facilities, he is a firm believer that we all need to get outside and exercise whenever possible, since outdoor exercise has many benefits, for both the body and the mind. http://www.Wholelifestyles.com

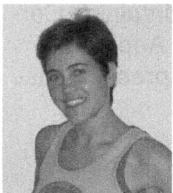

Beth Tascione, E-RYT 200, first experienced yoga as a four-year-old watching Lilias Folan on TV. It didn't take at that time, because her older brother would always sit she discovered yoga again as a stressed-out teenager in high school, where it wasn't exactly "cool" to do yoga. The third time was the charm: She turned to yoga as a respite in the middle of a hectic life juggling an acting career, "paying" work, married life and more. In 2003 she became a registered yoga instructor and is an advanced Relax and Renew Restorative Yoga Trainer. Beth teaches free outdoor yoga sessions in the summer as an offering to her community. She thinks it's a great way to build community and get outside and reconnect with nature. www.yogablissnyc.com

Notes from the Chapters

Notes from the Chapters

1. Selene Yeager, "Your Body's Biggest Enemy," *Women's Health*, Nov. 2009. This is an easy-to-understand summary of why sitting all day is so unhealthy. http://www.womenshealthmag.com/health/sedentary-lifestyle-hazards

2. John McKinney, "Thoreau Was Right: Nature Hones the Mind," Miller-McCune, January 11, 2011. This is a nifty little summary of how nature restores your mind. Available at:
http://www.miller-mccune.com/health/thoreau-was-right-nature-hones-the-mind-26763/

3. Thompson Coon J, et al., "Does participating in physical activity in outdoor natural environments have a greater effect on physical and mental wellbeing than physical activity indoors? A systematic review," *Environ Sci Technol,* 2011 Mar 1;45(5):1761-72. This is a technical paper that provides a summary of the benefits of exercising outdoors.

4. Jo Barton and Jules Pretty, "What is the Best Dose of Nature and Green Exercise for Improving Mental Health? A Multi-Study Analysis," Environ. Sci. Technol, 2010, 44 (10): 3947–3955.

5. Dr. Chi Pang Wen et al., "Minimum amount of physical activity for reduced mortality and extended life expectancy: a prospective cohort study," *The Lancet*, Early Online Publication, 16 August 2011doi:10.1016/S0140-6736(11)60749-6

6. "Quantity and Quality of Exercise for Developing and Maintaining Cardiorespiratory, Musculoskeletal, and Neuromotor Fitness in Apparently Healthy Adults: Guidance for Prescribing Exercise," ACSM press release June 2011. http://www.acsm.org.

7. Mayo Clinic. "Metabolism and weight loss: How you burn calories." http://www.mayoclinic.com/health/metabolism/WT00006

8. Jacob Liberman. *Light: Medicine of the Future* (Santa Fe, NM: Bear and Company, 1992).

9. Jennifer LaRue Huget, "Vitamin D: It's Necessary, but Getting Enough of It Is Not Necessarily Easy," Washington Post, May 12, 2009.

10. Frank Lipman, "Vitamin D: What You Need to Know," October 7, 2009, Huffington Post. http://www.huffingtonpost.com/dr-frank-lipman/vitamin-d-what-you-need-t_b_308973.html

Complementary Books

Colver, John. *Fit by Nature.* The Mountaineers Books, 2011.

Lauren, Mark. *You Are Your Own Gym.* Balantine Books, 2011.

Vindum, Tina. *Outdoor Fitness.* Falcon Guides, 2009.

Louv, Richard. *The Nature Principle: Human Restoration and the End of Nature-Deficit Disorder.* Algonquin Books, 2011.

Selhub, Eva M. and Logan, Alan C. *Your Brain On Nature: The Science of Nature's Influence on Your Health, Happiness and Vitality.* Wiley, 2012.

Yancey, Toni. *Instant Recess: Building a Fit Nation 10 Minutes at a Time* University of California Press, 2010.

The Fort Tryon Park Trust

The original DVD video that led to this book was sponsored by The Friends Committee of the Fort Tryon Park Trust. A portion of the proceeds from this book will go to the Trust. The Fort Tryon Park Trust's mission is to promote the restoration, preservation, and enhancement of this historic and scenic landmark for the benefit and use of the surrounding community and all New Yorkers. Please visit the Trust website, visit Fort Tryon Park, and support this marvelous organization, and enjoy this beautiful city park. http://www.FortTryonParkTrust.org

About the Author

About Nancy Bruning, CPT, MPH

Nancy Bruning is living the dream—but it took an *aha* moment. She was already a breast cancer survivor and author of over twenty-five books on health and fitness when she realized she was not following her own advice. There she sat, alone at her computer, hour after hour, with a bowl of Hershey's kisses to keep her awake and happy. She had a health club membership she didn't use as regularly as she wanted. She was not taking full advantage of her neighborhood parks. She decided to integrate exercise, people, and science into a healthier life by becoming a certified personal trainer and earning a master's degree in public health. Today Nancy is a certified Physical Activity Professional in Public Health Specialist (American College of Sport Medicine). Nancercize offers outdoor exercise classes for groups and individual clients in New York City parks and recreation areas, as well as other parts of the US. Nancy also trains others in outdoor fitness techniques so they can lead their own groups. Her popular weight management program, scientifically sound and backed by her own extensive research and experience, offers an entire lifestyle makeover.

Visit Nancy's website, Nancercize.net to find out more about Nancercize outdoor exercise classes for groups and individuals, trainings for professionals and regular folk, wellness and weight loss programs, her appearances and speaking engagements, as well as Nancy's 25 previous books on wellness, weight loss, and natural therapies.

Connect with her at nancy@nancercize.net or 419-962-6292. She's waiting and ready for you to ask her how to start a Nancercize program in a park near you!

Talk with Nancy on Twitter: http://twitter.com/nancercize
Like her Updates on Facebook: http://www.facebook.com/Nancercize
Listen to her internet radio show: http://www.blogtalkradio.com/nancercize
Watch her video: http://www.youtube.com/Nancercize